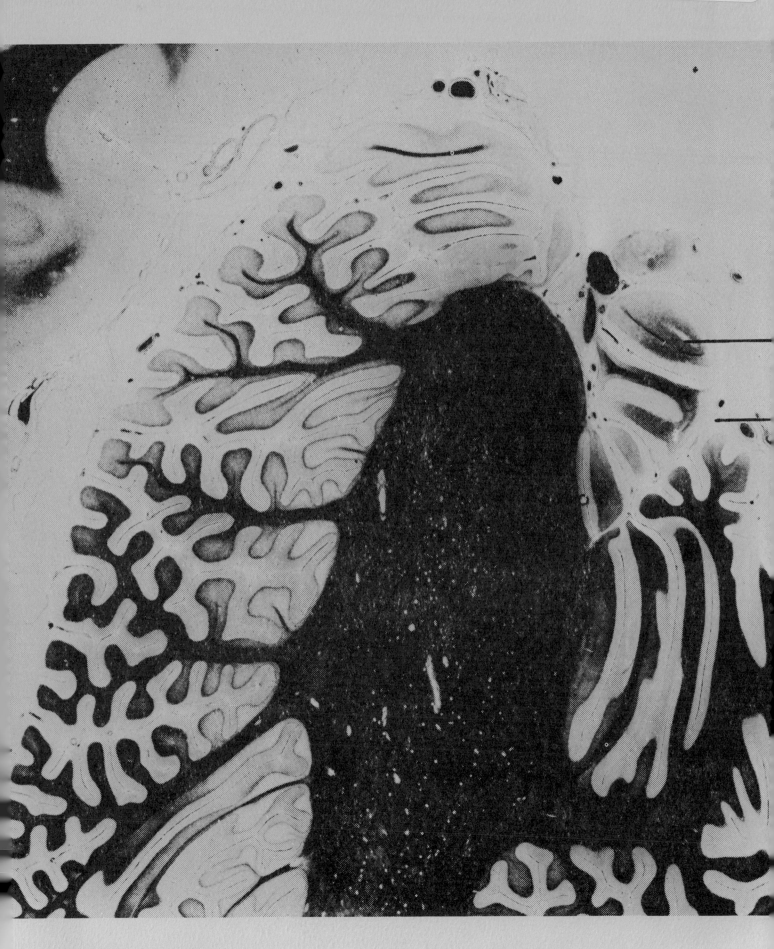

ATLAS OF THE

Central Nervous System in Man

Second Edition

ATLAS OF THE
Central Nervous

The Williams & Wilkins Company
BALTIMORE

System in Man

second edition

Richard A. Miller, B.S., M.S., Ph.D.

Professor of Anatomy, Neil Hellman Research Building,
Albany Medical College, Union University

Ethel Burack, A.B., Ph.D., M.D.

Associate Professor of Anatomy, Neil Hellman Research Building,
Albany Medical College, Union University

Made in the United States of America

First Edition, 1968
Reprinted 1968
Reprinted 1969
Reprinted 1973
Reprinted 1974

Library of Congress Cataloging in Publication Data

Miller, Richard Avery, 1911–
   Atlas of the central nervous system in man.

   Includes indexes.
   1. Central nervous system—Atlases. 2. Neuroan-
atomy—Atlases. I. Burack, Ethel, 1907–joint author.
II. Title. [DNLM: 1. Central nervous system—
Anatomy and histology—Atlases. WL17 M649a]
QM451.M53   611'.81'0222   1976-21054
ISBN 0-683-06127-5

Composed and Printed at
Waverly Press, Inc.
Mt. Royal and Guilford Aves.
Baltimore, Md. 21202, U.S.A.

CONTENTS

PREFACE TO THE SECOND EDITION

Twenty-one of the original Weigert sections, cut transversely were rephotographed for this second edition. In two instances this was done purely for technical reasons. However, among the valued comments from users of the first edition was the suggestion that the spinal cord and lower brain stem could be enlarged to a greater size. Accordingly, in this edition, sections of the spinal cord are enlarged 14 times. Most of the cerebellum was cropped from Figures 7 through 13 inclusive, and sections of the medulla are magnified 8 times, twice the original enlargement. So as to retain the deep cerebellar nuclei and the course of the inferior cerebellar peduncle, Figures 14 and 15 are 5-fold enlargements. The magnification of Figures 16 to 19 is 7 times. The balance of the transverse figures and all sagittal figures are enlarged 4 times and 3.4 times, respectively. All of the structures identified in the first edition are still labeled here.

Almost all of the explanations of figures have been revised. The most extensive changes, particularly of those annotations pertaining to the transverse sections, reflect changes in conceptions and

information since the preparation of the original publication. Some changes are nominal.

The nomenclature continues to be that of the Paris Nomina Anatomica (1955). Few if any of the terms applicable to this atlas that were approved at the International Congresses of Anatomists in 1960 and 1965 are used in the current editions of the textbooks of neuroanatomy published in this country.

Thirty-five millimeter color transparencies of the Weigert slides used in the atlas, but without labeling, were released in 1973. These sections also have been photographed anew. The new set reflects the greater enlargement of the transverse sections in the atlas but are not identical with them. In transparencies of Figures 23 to 38, for example, the vertical format was adopted; this permits inclusion of somewhat more than the right half of the sections and at greater enlargement than was possible in the atlas. The color transparencies in the sagittal series are of sections all of which, rather than some, were counterstained in Congo red. They correspond in every other way to Figures 39 to 63.

PREFACE TO THE FIRST EDITION

This atlas is dedicated to the memory of Dr. Robert Sydney Cunningham, who became professor of anatomy, chairman of the Department of Anatomy, and Dean of the Albany Medical College in 1937 and who later assumed additional responsibility as administrator of the Albany Hospital. His pioneering efforts in the development of both institutions laid the groundwork for what is now the Albany Medical Center. However, Dr. Cunningham was also a remarkable teacher, and it was this phase of his activities that he found most enjoyable. He was well aware of the value of excellent teaching material. More immediately, Dr. Cunningham appreciated the importance of myelin-stained sections, cut in sagittal as well as transverse planes, in the acquisition of that thorough command of the organization of the nervous system which is basic to the skillful use of the clinical neurologic examination. Moreover, Dr. Cunningham had the requisite knowledge and skill to obtain complete serial sections of two brains with major

vessels intact that were well preserved, well cut and mounted, and well stained, no small feat indeed.

Basically, the annotations are a commitment to paper of one aspect of the course in neuroanatomy as it has been taught since 1950, although the Weigert slides have been used here since 1940. The Weigert sections, which are mounted as standard lantern slides, are projected on a screen and used as a basis for discussion with and quizzing of medical students. In these sessions the origin, course, termination, anatomic relations, blood supply, and function of fiber tracts and nuclei are correlated with their visual images, so that an integrated concept of structure and function is gradually achieved. The neuroanatomic bases of the more common neurologic problems are also brought out. The numerous cross references to other levels of transverse and sagittal series made possible by the format of an atlas greatly facilitate appreciation of the anatomic relationships.

The notes, particularly those to the transverse

figures, attempt to develop a concept of the functional organization of the central nervous system by a running account of segmental reflex pathways and of suprasegmental fiber tracts to and from higher levels of the central nervous system. The notes are purposely kept simple and controversial material is avoided. The practice of indicating both the origin and the termination of each major fiber tract (by cross references) when it first appears in the illustrations and relating it to function seems to facilitate an earlier conceptualization of the nervous system.

The annotations also attempt to develop concepts in three dimensions of the structural organization of the central nervous system. This aspect receives major emphasis, along with the blood supply of the brain stem, in the annotations of the sagittal figures.

The labeling of structures in the figures is more complete than most initial courses in neuroanatomy today would require. The intent here was both to satisfy the curiosity of observant medical students and to make the atlas useful to those who desire more than the fundamentals provided by the annotations.

For the most part, the nomenclature of the Paris revision of the BNA has been used. Ordinarily, the English equivalents are employed except where the Latin is vernacular. This seemed justified in what was planned primarily as an atlas for students.

The authors have a multiple indebtedness to Dr. J. M. Wolfe, who followed Dr. Cunningham as chairman of the Anatomy Department, not only because he was among those (along with one of us, E. B.) who skillfully differentiated the Weigert slides, but primarily because he generously permitted these sections to be used for this atlas and because he assigned us with unrestricted freedom to the course in which the annotations were conceived.

Miss Patricia Lynch has been remarkably cheerful, always patient, and everlastingly careful in typing the manuscript.

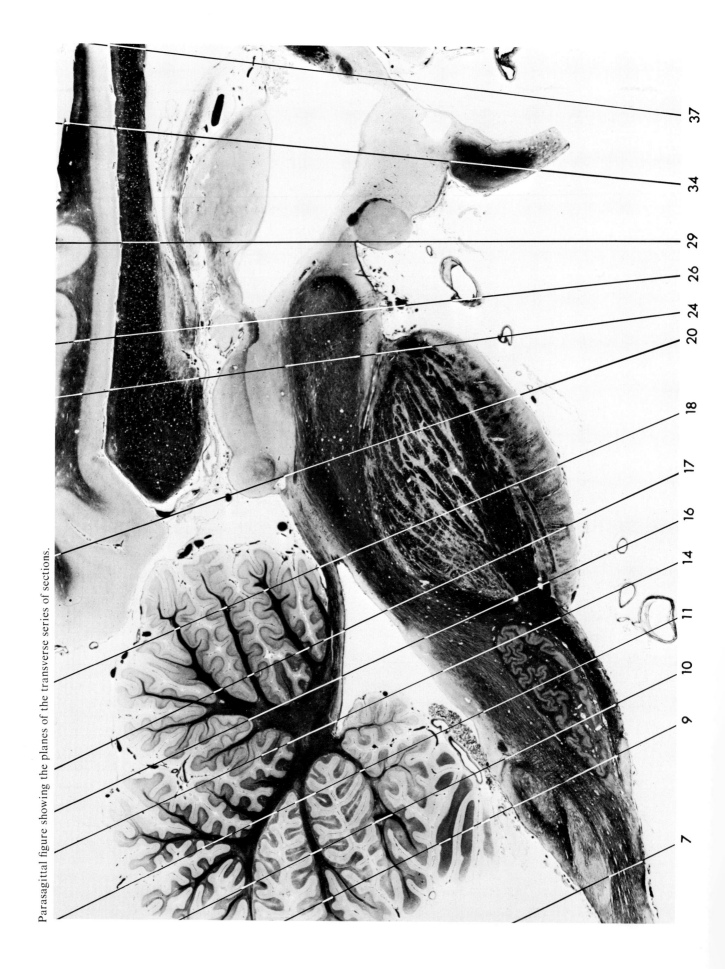

Parasagittal figure showing the planes of the transverse series of sections.

TRANSVERSE

INTRODUCTION TO THE

This initial segment of the atlas consists of 6 representative levels of the spinal cord and 32 levels of the brain cut transversely in the medulla and lower pons, with a gradual shift to frontal sections beginning in the rostral pons and progressing into the thalamus and cerebral hemispheres.

The planes of representative transverse sections are indicated in the sagittal section on a preceding page, and are numbered 7 to 37, denoting Figures 7 to 37. This parasagittal section (actually a duplicate of Fig. 44) was selected because it shows such important landmarks as the inferior olive, abducens nucleus, inferior and superior colliculi, mamillary body, and red nucleus. These structures, which are not visible in a midsagittal section, are important in delimiting the five major subdivisions of the brain from myelencephalon to telencephalon. The small numbers at the top of each of the representative transverse figures (Figs. 7 to 37) indicate the planes of selected sagittal figures. Their usage is discussed in the "Introduction to the Sagittal Plates" (following Fig. 38).

Structures are identified by code numbers so as to make possible the use of large illustrations in a book of reasonable proportions. Moreover, this system has an added advantage in that it makes possible a form of programmed instruction with immediate feedback when a legend is consulted. The code is based upon the sagittal sections. Beginning with Figure 39 and continuing in successive parasagittal sections, structures in the medulla were numbered between 1 and 99; pontine structures were numbered in the 100's, mesencephalic structures in the 200's, diencephalic derivatives in the 300's, and telencephalic derivatives in the 400's. Letters were used to identify structures in-

TRANSVERSE FIGURES

digenous to the spinal cord alone. Thus, the numbering of fiber tracts and blood vessels which extend longitudinally for some distance in the central nervous system was determined by the segment of the brain in which a structure first appeared in the sagittal sections. However, for most nuclei, some fiber tracts, and some blood vessels, the number locates the structure's position within one of the five major subdivisions of the brain. This frequently delimits the area of a figure which must be searched to locate a desired structure, particularly in the sagittal figures, but also in rostral transverse or frontal sections where parts of the pons, mesencephalon, thalamus, and cerebral hemispheres may all be represented.

Generally the names used are those adopted or suggested in the Paris revision of the BNA. The names have been translated into English, except where the Latin is commonly retained. In translating, adjectives were uniformly placed before the noun in the reverse of the Latin order, so that the major modifier immediately precedes the noun. For example, the nucleus ventralis anterior becomes anterior ventral nucleus. This is the accepted practice except for thalamic nuclei, where the order of adjectives is not consistently reversed by some writers.

Structures which appear in a consecutive series of figures are usually labeled only in every other plate. Thus, although every structure labeled in a figure is listed in its legend, the annotations may refer to nuclei or fibers which are labeled only in the plate that precedes or follows.

Two indices are provided: in addition to the alphabetical index, structures are also indexed in the numerical order of their code numbers.

FIGURE 1. Sacral Spinal Cord

This first page of comment deals primarily with general features which are characteristic of all levels of the spinal cord, not just of the sacral portion. The spinal cord is surrounded by the posterior (A) and anterior (F) roots of spinal nerves. The cell bodies of fibers in the posterior roots, here and at other levels of the cord, are located in posterior root ganglia which are not included in these sections. The large, heavily myelinated fibers of a posterior root enter the spinal cord and divide into ascending and descending branches in the gracile fasciculus (2); ascending fibers may rise as far as the gracile nucleus (3, Fig. 8) before synapse, but some synapse in the posterior horn and never reach the gracile nucleus. Descending fibers in the gracile fasciculus synapse within one or two segments of entry.

Similarly, the fine, lightly myelinated fibers of a posterior root enter lateral to the large fibers and bifurcate in the dorsolateral fasciculus (B). Ascending branches ascend no more than five segments before synapsing in the substantia gelatinosa (C) or nucleus proprius in the dorsal horn (H). Most fibers ascending in the dorsolateral fasciculus synapse close to the level of entry. Descending fibers are always short, and they synapse in the dorsal horn within one or two segments of entry.

The cell bodies of the axons contained in an anterior root are located in the anterior horn (J). Large perikarya give rise to the large myelinated alpha efferent fibers in the anterior root which innervate skeletal muscle; small neurons give origin to the gamma efferent fibers which innervate the intrafusal muscle fibers in muscle spindles of skeletal muscles. Neurons of an intermediate size at sacral levels (parasympathetic nucleus (I)) give rise to parasympathetic, preganglionic fibers in sacral spinal nerves 2, 3, and 4. Similar neurons

in the intermediolateral nucleus (N, Figs. 4 and 5) in the thoracic and the upper two lumbar segments give rise to sympathetic, preganglionic fibers.

In some instances, primary afferent fibers in posterior roots synapse directly upon alpha efferent neurons, but more commonly one or more neurons are interposed between afferent and efferent neurons. When these internuncial neurons are confined to the spinal cord, their axons are said to be intra- or intersegmental fibers. The cell bodies of such fibers are generally located in the posterior horn, and their axons ascend or descend in the white matter of the cord close to the gray matter in the fasciculi proprii (D) of the lateral, anterior, and posterior funiculi.

Fibers of secondary neurons which ascend through the spinal cord and enter the brain stem are called suprasegmental fibers. Groups of such fibers form the long ascending tracts; their cell bodies are located in the posterior horn. Although they may give rise to collateral fibers in their ascent, the terminal synapse is always in the brain. More specifically, they are afferent suprasegmental fibers, since they convey nerve impulses initiated in peripheral receptors and propagated in primary neurons contained in posterior roots to the ascending tract.

The cell bodies of suprasegmental efferent fibers are located in various nuclei in the brain. They form long descending suprasegmental tracts in the spinal cord and synapse on alpha and gamma efferent neurons, either directly or via intrasegmental, internuncial neurons. The most important of these are the lateral corticospinal (37), vestibulospinal (35), and reticulospinal (K) tracts.

Thus, there are three classes of fibers coursing rostrocaudally in the white matter of the spinal cord: primary afferent fibers (gracile

fasciculus, dorsolateral fasciculus), inter- and intrasegmental fibers (fasciculi proprii), and suprasegmental fibers (long ascending and descending fiber tracts). The major suprasegmental afferent and suprasegmental efferent fiber tracts of the sacral spinal cord are identified in this figure, but will be discussed later.

A—Posterior roots
B—Dorsolateral fasciculus
C—Substantia gelatinosa
D—Fasciculi proprii
E—Spinoreticular tract
F—Anterior roots
G—Posterior root fibers
H—Nucleus proprius of the posterior horn
I—Parasympathetic nucleus
J—Anterior horn
K—Reticulospinal tract
2—Gracile fasciculus
33—Anterior spinocerebellar tract
35—Vestibulospinal tract
37—Lateral corticospinal tract
38—Anterior spinothalamic tract
133—Lateral spinothalamic tract

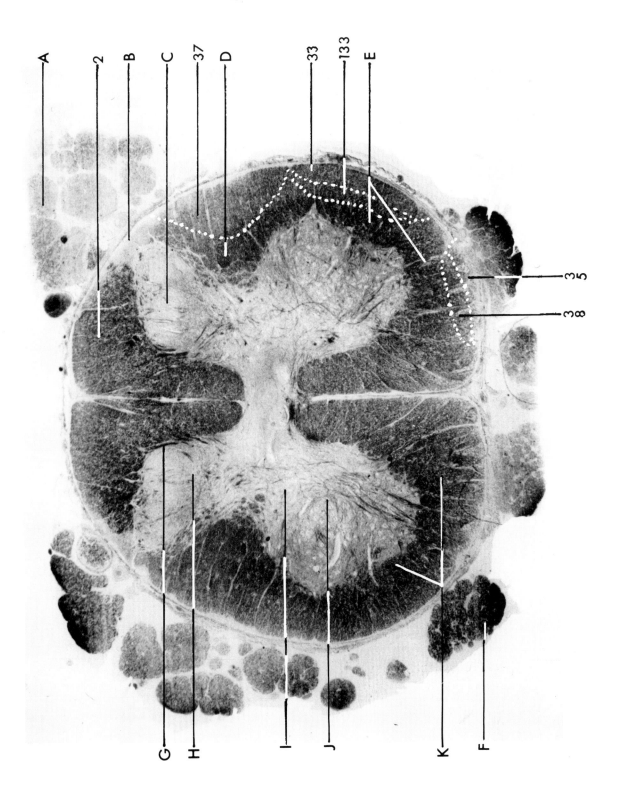

1

FIGURE 2. Lower Lumbar Spinal Cord

Comment here is directed chiefly to the long ascending and descending tracts in the spinal cord at this level. Two major parts of the posterior horn which are easily distinguished in Weigert sections are the substantia gelatinosa (C) and the nucleus proprius (H). Neurons in these two nuclear groups are intercalated between primary neurons and those which give origin to some of the long ascending tracts, the so called secondary neurons. The sites of perikarya that give rise to most of the large ascending tracts are somewhat uncertain. Available evidence suggests they are located ventral of the nucleus proprius in the intermediate area formed by the bases of posterior and anterior (J) horns.

One ascending tract of secondary fibers, the anterior spinocerebellar tract (33), occupies the perimeter of the lateral funiculus immediately anterior of the lateral corticospinal tract (37). It arises in neurons of the intermediate area; most axons cross in the anterior white commissure (Q) to join a few uncrossed fibers at the edge of the spinal cord (Figs. 1 to 6) and medulla oblongata (Figs. 7 to 14). In the pons (Fig. 16), the tract enters the cerebellum via the superior cerebellar peduncle where it recrosses the midline and terminates in the cortex of the anterior lobe (Fig. 39), ipsilateral with its origin.

Impulses in this tract produce no sensation but, instead, participate in the reflex adjustments of the inferior extremities. The receptive endings of primary fibers which monosynaptically excite the anterior spinocerebellar tract are Golgi tendon receptors in muscles of the legs and lower part of the body.

The lateral spinothalamic tract (133) lies in part medial to and in part intermingles with the anterior spinocerebellar fibers. This tract originates in the intermediate area of the spinal cord throughout its length. The fibers cross in the anterior white commissure (Q). The first fibers to cross at sacral levels occupy a position closest to the lateral corticospinal tract (37). Fibers conveying impulses initiated in more rostral dermatomes and crossing at successively higher levels join the lateral spinothalamic tract in layers along its medial and anterior aspect. The terminal fibers of the tract synapse in the posterolateral ventral thalamic nucleus (336, Fig. 28).

The peripheral receptors of the primary fibers which convey impulses to these spinothalamic fibers are those excited particularly by painful and thermal stimuli. The fibers are the fine, lightly myelinated components of the posterior roots (A) which ascend and descend briefly in the dorsolateral fasciculus (B), before synapsing upon internuncial neurons in the posterior horn (C, H) which convey impulses to those neurons of the intermediate area that initiate the lateral spinothalamic tract. The impulses upon reaching the thalamus are perceived as pain and temperature.

The large myelinated primary fibers with peripheral receptors which are excited particularly by light tactile stimuli enter and bifurcate into branches that ascend and descend in the gracile fasciculus (2) before some of those posterior root fibers (G) enter the nucleus proprius (H). Presumably there is an intercalated neuron that conveys impulses to neurons in the intermediate area which give origin to secondary fibers that also cross in the anterior white commissure (Q) and then turn rostrally as the anterior spinothalamic tract (38) along the perimeter of the anterior funiculus. This tract also ultimately terminates in the posterolateral ventral thalamic nucleus. A tactile receptor also has synaptic connections in the spinal cord and brain stem which mediate reflexes.

At all levels in the anterior part of the lateral funiculus and in the anterior funiculus between the spinothalamic tracts and the fasciculi proprii (D) are spinoreticular fibers (E), named for their origin and destination. They have not yet been delineated by anatomical procedures, but are known to play an important part in maintaining consciousness.

Of the long descending suprasegmental tracts which occur at this and at sacral levels, the lateral corticospinal tract (37) is preeminent. The cell bodies of these fibers are located in circumscribed areas of the cerebral cortex. Corticospinal fibers are constituents of the internal capsule (418, Fig. 35); they occupy the middle portion of each crus cerebri (220, Fig. 25), extend throughout sections of the basilar pons (Figs. 23 to 16), and form the pyramids of the medulla (14, Figs. 14 to 8), where they are also labeled corticospinal fibers (118). These fibers synapse in the spinal cord and directly or indirectly excite the motor neurons in the anterior horn which supply skeletal musculature. They facilitate tone of muscle and effect the fine, discrete volitional movements of the body.

The vestibulospinal tract (35) arises in the lateral vestibular nucleus (143, Fig. 14). The fibers, which descend ipsilaterally to synapse indirectly and directly upon alpha efferent neurons, are important in reflex adjustments of the body and in the maintenance of tone in skeletal muscles.

Reticulospinal fibers (K) arise in the reticular formation of the mesencephalon, pons, and medulla (34, Fig. 12), and occupy as yet undefined regions in the anterior and anterolateral portions of the spinal cord. They modulate volitional movements and skeletal muscular tonus, and mediate reflexes involving smooth muscle and glands.

A—Posterior roots
B—Dorsolateral fasciculus
C—Substantia gelatinosa
D—Fasciculi proprii
E—Spinoreticular tract
F—Anterior roots
G—Posterior root fibers
H—Nucleus proprius of the posterior horn
J—Anterior horn
K—Reticulospinal tract
Q—Anterior white commissure
T—Posterior spinal artery
U—Anterior spinal artery
2—Gracile fasciculus
33—Anterior spinocerebellar tract
35—Vestibulospinal tract
37—Lateral corticospinal tract
38—Anterior spinothalamic tract
133—Lateral spinothalamic tract

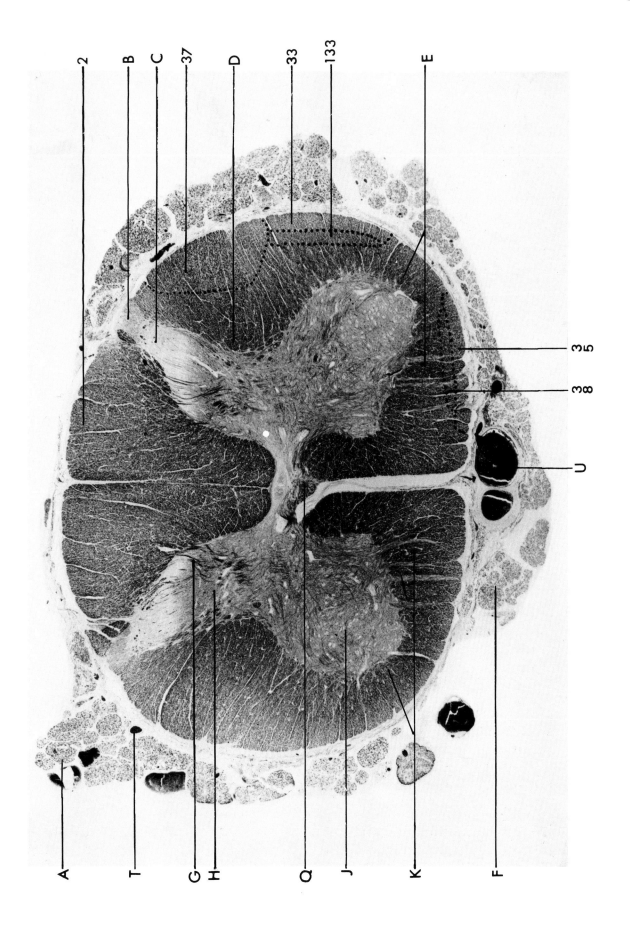

FIGURE 3. Upper Lumbar Spinal Cord

Figures 1 and 2 represent transverse levels in the lumbosacral enlargement. In these the anterior horn of the gray matter is large because there are many alpha and gamma motor neurons related to the innervation of the inferior extremity; likewise, the posterior gray horn is massive because of the large influx of primary afferent fibers from the skin of the inferior extremity, pelvis, and buttocks. At upper lumbar levels the area of gray matter is diminished because it is related to an abdominal area, with less musculature and skin than the inferior extremity. In contrast, the amount of white matter is greater here than in Figures 1 and 2 because suprasegmental descending fibers progressively leave the white matter and synapse in the gray matter, while suprasegmental ascending fibers accumulate progressively at ever higher levels of the spinal cord.

It is generally true that most of the long ascending tracts are present throughout the spinal cord. One major exception is the posterior spinocerebellar tract. This tract is also exceptional in that the nucleus of origin is known to be the dorsal nucleus (M) or Clarke's column. It appears as a medial bulge of the posterior gray horn into the dorsal funiculus. In view of the fact that the dorsal nucleus does not occur below L2 (or above T1), only a few fibers of the posterior spinocerebellar tract could already have reached the ipsilateral perimeter of the lateral funiculus between the dorsolateral fasciculus (B) and the anterior spinocerebellar tract (33); accordingly, none are indicated in this figure. The posterior spinocerebellar tract becomes a tract of appreciable size at higher levels (24, Figs. 4 to 6). The dorsal nucleus receives impulses initiated in receptors located in muscles, joints, (and tendons) in the lower part of the body and conducted by large primary fibers. Those fast conducting primary fibers which enter the spinal cord below L2 ascend in the fasciculus

gracilis (Figs. 1 and 2) to reach and synapse in the caudal end of the dorsal nucleus. The posterior spinocerebellar tract terminates ipsilaterally in the anterior and posterior vermis of the cerebellum, entering via the inferior cerebellar peduncle (28, Fig. 14). Like the anterior spinocerebellar tract, it conveys neural information to the cerebellum which enables it to modulate the reflex adjustments of the body.

Several small tracts of more or less unknown function occupy the area at the perimeter of the spinal cord where the anterior roots emerge in the anterolateral sulcus (L) at the junction of the lateral and anterior funiculi. Fibers of the spinotectal tract originate at all levels of the spinal cord in the contralateral posterior horn (H), and terminate in the superior colliculus (210, Fig. 23). An alternative view is that collateral axons of lateral spinothalamic fibers synapse in the superior colliculus and that there is no discrete spinotectal tract. Spino-olivary and olivospinal tracts also occupy this general area. Spino-olivary fibers occur at all levels of the spinal cord. It has been suggested that the spino-olivary tract conveys impulses initiated in those cutaneous receptors sensitive to tactile stimuli, but this is not an established fact; the impulses ultimately reach the cerebellum via olivocerebellar fibers and the inferior cerebellar peduncle (27 and 28, Fig. 14).

B—Dorsolateral fasciculus
C—Substantia gelatinosa
D—Fasciculi proprii
E—Spinoreticular tract
H—Nucleus proprius of the posterior horn
K—Reticulospinal tract
L—Anterolateral sulcus
M—Dorsal nucleus
Q—Anterior white commissure
2—Gracile fasciculus
33—Anterior spinocerebellar tract
35—Vestibulospinal tract
37—Lateral corticospinal tract
38—Anterior spinothalamic tract
133—Lateral spinothalamic tract

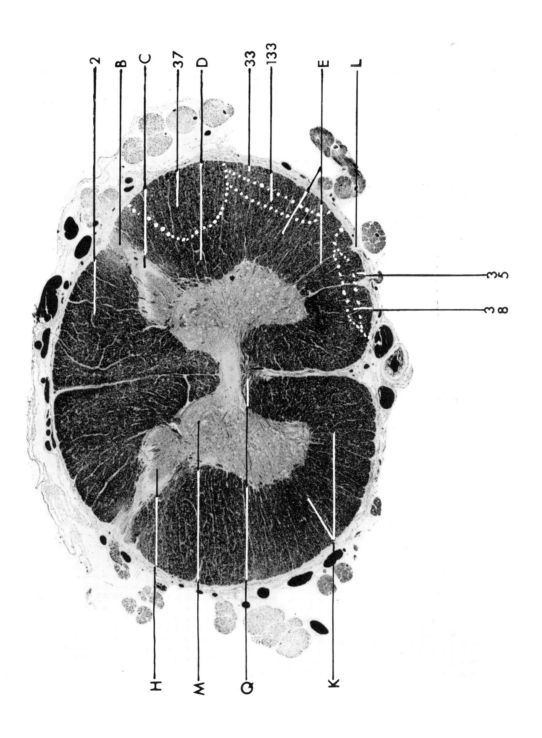

FIGURE 4. Lower Thoracic Spinal Cord

Even though the spinal cord is appreciably smaller here than at the levels of the lumbosacral enlargement (Figs. 1 and 2), it is obvious that the diminution is due to the reduced area of gray matter rather than to a reduction of white matter. Indeed, the area of the dorsal, lateral, and anterior funicular white matter is actually greater than at lower levels of the spinal cord. This is a result of the progressive accumulation of ascending suprasegmental fibers, in addition to a greater number of descending fibers that extend to lower levels of the spinal cord. There is, moreover, one new descending tract, the rubrospinal (40), which in man does not extend below the thoracic segments of the spinal cord. This tract arises in the red nucleus (214, Fig. 25) and crosses in the ventral tegmental decussation (224, Fig. 24). It appears to be one of the minor tracts in man, as it is smaller in man than in animals. In animals, impulses conducted in the tract facilitate tone and activity in flexor muscles. It characteristically occupies a position in the angle formed by the lateral corticospinal tract dorsally and the anterior spinocerebellar tract laterally. It has been suggested that reticulospinal (K) fibers may be assuming the functions of the rubrospinal tract.

A nucleus coextensive with the nucleus dorsalis (M) between T1 and L2 is the intermediolateral nucleus (N), so called because it forms a lateral projection of gray matter between the anterior (J) and posterior (H) horns. It is the source of preganglionic fibers to the sympathetic chain ganglia and collateral ganglia of the sympathetic division of the autonomic nervous system.

B—Dorsolateral fasciculus
C—Substantia gelatinosa
D—Fasciculi proprii
E—Spinoreticular tract
H—Nucleus proprius of the posterior horn
J—Anterior horn
K—Reticulospinal tract
M—Dorsal nucleus
N—Intermediolateral nucleus
2—Gracile fasciculus
24—Posterior spinocerebellar tract
33—Anterior spinocerebellar tract
35—Vestibulospinal tract
37—Lateral corticospinal tract
38—Anterior spinothalamic tract
40—Rubrospinal tract
133—Lateral spinothalamic tract

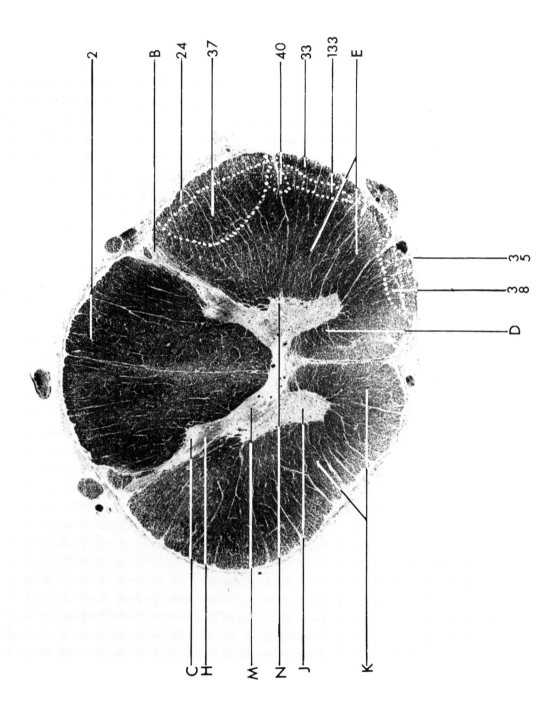

FIGURE 5. Upper Thoracic Spinal Cord

At the upper thoracic levels the spinal cord is distinctly oval in cross section, whereas it is roughly quadrangular at sacral levels and round at the lower thoracic and upper lumbar portions. Shape is only one characteristic which identifies the upper thoracic spinal cord. The posterior funiculus, which is wholly occupied with the gracile fasciculus at levels below T6, now is divided by a posterior intermediate septum (R) into a medial, gracile fasciculus (2) and a lateral, cuneate fasciculus (20). Just as those large primary fibers of nerves below T6 ascend in laminar array lateral of the posterior median septum (V), so those of nerves above T6 accumulate in laminar array, parallel with the posterior intermediate septum in the cuneate fasciculus (20). Many of the primary fibers in the cuneate fasciculus ascend into the medulla oblongata and synapse in the cuneate nucleus (21, Fig. 9), where the impulses are relayed by secondary fibers to the thalamus. The sensory components of the cuneate fasciculus, like those of the gracile fasciculus, are concerned with tactile and positional sensibility. However, where the gracile fasciculus conveys impulses initiated in the inferior extremity and the lower part of the body, the cuneate fasciculus is related to the upper part of the body and the superior extremity.

Several descending fiber tracts that do not extend into the lower part of the spinal cord are present in the anterior funiculus on either side of the anterior median fissure (S). The anterior corticospinal tract (1), closest to the fissure, has the same origin as the lateral corticospinal tract (37) and courses with it from the cerebral cortex to the level of the pyramidal decussation. At the decussation (4, Fig. 7) the anterior corticospinal tract continues uncrossed straight into the spinal cord. In the spinal cord some of the fibers cross in the anterior white commissure (Q), while others remain uncrossed to their terminal synapse in the anterior horn. Usually, a small neuron is

interposed between a corticospinal fiber and the motor neuron innervating the skeletal muscle.

Lateral to the anterior corticospinal tract is the medial longitudinal fasciculus (8). The tract contains some of the descending fibers of the medial longitudinal fasciculus and tectospinal tract in the brain stem (8 and 9, Figs. 25 to 8 and 39). Some of the fibers arise from cell bodies located in the medial vestibular nucleus (128, Figs. 14 to 11), superior colliculus (210, Fig. 21), and interstitial nucleus (225, Fig. 23). Most of these fibers terminate in the anterior gray matter of the cervical enlargement, but a few are present in the upper thoracic levels. Probably they are concerned with reflex postural adjustments, particularly of the upper extremity, in response to vestibular and optic stimuli.

B—Dorsolateral fasciculus
C—Substantia gelatinosa
E—Spinoreticular tract
H—Nucleus proprius of the posterior horn
K—Reticulospinal tract
M—Dorsal nucleus
N—Intermediolateral nucleus
P—Dentate ligament
Q—Anterior white commissure
R—Posterior intermediate septum
S—Anterior median fissure
V—Posterior median septum
1—Anterior corticospinal tract
2—Gracile fasciculus
8—Medial longitudinal fasciculus
20—Cuneate fasciculus
24—Posterior spinocerebellar tract
33—Anterior spinocerebellar tract
35—Vestibulospinal tract
37—Lateral corticospinal tract
38—Anterior spinothalamic tract
40—Rubrospinal tract
133—Lateral spinothalamic tract

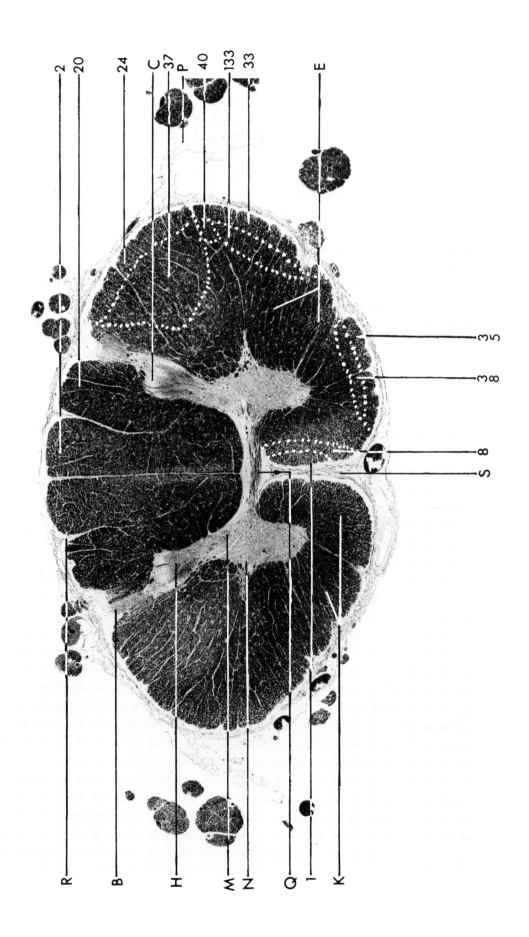

FIGURE 6. Cervical Enlargement, Spinal Cord

In general configuration, the cervical enlargement resembles the upper thoracic segment in most respects. However, since the cervical enlargement gives origin to motor fibers of the brachial plexus and receives its afferent fibers, the posterior and anterior horns of gray matter are large. The lateral bulges of the anterior gray matter, which clearly help to swell the section into its oval shape, contain the alpha and gamma efferent neurons innervating the skeletal muscles of the upper extremity. Two columns of neurons, present in the previous section, are absent from the cervical portion of the spinal cord: the intermediolateral cell column and the dorsal nucleus. Hence, sympathetic preganglionic fibers and posterior spinocerebellar fibers do not originate in the cervical region. A few anterior spinocerebellar fibers may arise and be added to the tract here. However, many of the impulses from receptors in the muscles, joints, (and tendons) in the upper extremity reach the cerebellum via a different series of neurons, to wit: central processes of large, myelinated primary fibers ascend in the cuneate fasciculus (20) of the cervical cord and synapse in the accessory cuneate nucleus (44, Fig. 9), from which secondary axons enter the inferior cerebellar peduncle (28, Fig. 10) to ascend into the cerebellum.

The volume of white matter in all funiculi is very great in the cervical spinal cord because, in addition to many inter- and intrasegmental fibers in the fasciculi proprii (D), the funiculi now contain all the sup
rasegmental tracts ascending into the brain from the spinal cord, as well as all descending from the brain to the spinal cord.

B—Dorsolateral fasciculus
C—Substantia gelatinosa
D—Fasciculi proprii
E- Spinoreticular tract
H—Nucleus proprius of the posterior horn
K—Reticulospinal tract
Q—Anterior white commissure
R—Posterior intermediate septum
1—Anterior corticospinal tract
2—Gracile fasciculus
8—Medial longitudinal fasciculus
20—Cuneate fasciculus
24—Posterior spinocerebellar tract
33—Anterior spinocerebellar tract
35—Vestibulospinal tract
37—Lateral corticospinal tract
38—Anterior spinothalamic tract
40—Rubrospinal tract
133—Lateral spinothalamic tract

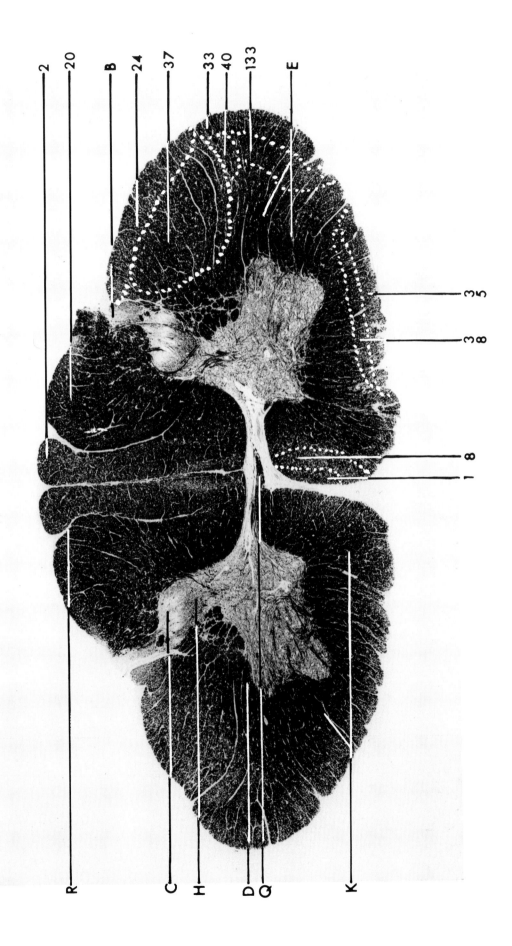

FIGURE 7. Pyramidal Decussation, Medulla Oblongata

The figure shows the lowermost end of the medulla oblongata, close to its junction with the spinal cord. As might be anticipated, most of the ascending and descending tracts occupy positions similar to those they occupy in the spinal cord. The figure shows the lower end of the decussation of the pyramids (4), in which corticospinal fibers cross over to the opposite side of the medulla. Pyramid is the gross anatomical name for the corticospinal fibers in the medulla (14, Figs. 9 and 40). In this decussation of the pyramids, corticospinal fibers extend both dorsally and laterally to achieve their position as the lateral corticospinal tract (37) in the spinal cord (Figs. 6 to 1). Some fibers do not cross, but extend into the cord where as the anterior corticospinal tract (1) they continue to occupy a ventral parasagittal position. In addition, a few pyramidal fibers remain uncrossed but move dorsally and mingle with the crossed lateral corticospinal fibers.

In contrast to the fiber tracts, the configuration of the gray matter is appreciably changed, however. Although an anterior gray horn (J) is still recognizable, the positions of the posterior gray horn and the dorsolateral fasciculus are now occupied by the spinal trigeminal nucleus (19) and the spinal trigeminal tract (25). The spinal trigeminal tract consists of primary fibers whose cell bodies are chiefly contained in the trigeminal ganglion and whose peripheral processes are related to those receptors in the face which are excited by painful and thermal stimuli. The central processes of these primary neurons penetrate the brain at the midpontine level (150, Fig. 16). Some of the fibers accumulate and course inferiorly as the spinal trigeminal tract; this tract can be followed in all the intervening sections of the brain stem (25, Figs. 16 to 7) into the upper cervical portion of the spinal cord, where they interdigitate with ascending fibers in the dorsolateral fasciculus. Many of

the fibers of the spinal trigeminal tract, however, do not descend into the spinal cord but, instead, synapse on secondary neurons which also extend as a long column of cells from midpontine levels to the spinal cord. This column is the spinal trigeminal nucleus (19). It is always located immediately medial to the spinal trigeminal tract. The spinal trigeminal nucleus gives origin to secondary fibers, some of which mediate reflexes. Others, which ascend into the thalamus as suprasegmental afferent fibers, convey impulses which are perceived as painful, thermal, and possibly tactile sensations in the face.

There are also a few general somatic afferent fibers in cranial nerves VII, IX, and X. Their peripheral receptors, located in the ear and Eustachian tube, are activated by painful stimuli; the central processes of these primary neurons are also components of the spinal trigeminal tract and synapse in the spinal trigeminal nucleus. Thus, all painful and thermal stimuli originating in the face are mediated by the spinal trigeminal tract and nucleus.

J—Anterior horn
1—Anterior corticospinal tract
2—Gracile fasciculus
4—Decussation of the pyramids
19—Spinal trigeminal nucleus
20—Cuneate fasciculus
24—Posterior spinocerebellar tract
25—Spinal tract of the trigeminal nerve
33—Anterior spinocerebellar tract
35—Vestibulospinal tract
37—Lateral corticospinal tract
38—Anterior spinothalamic tract
40—Rubrospinal tract
108—Tonsil
133—Lateral spinothalamic tract

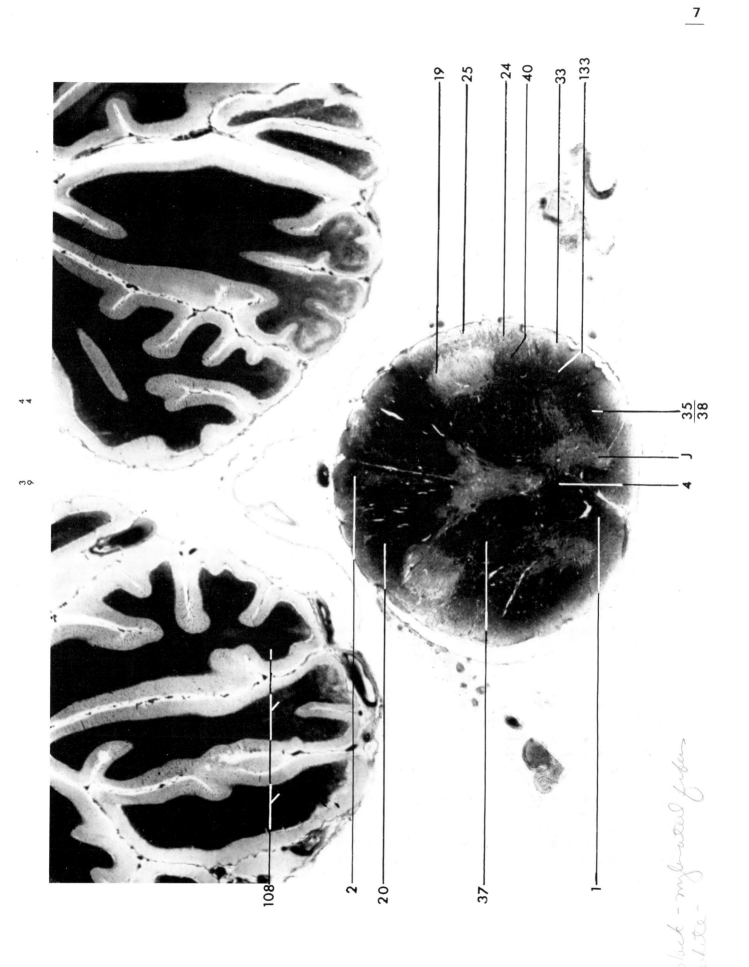

19

25

24

40

33

133

35
—
38

J

4

44

39

108

2

20

37

1

black - myelinated fiber
white -

FIGURE 8. Medulla Oblongata, Pyramidal Decussation

Since the plane of this figure passes through the rostral end of the decussation of the corticospinal fibers (118), the lateral and anterior corticospinal tracts are not visible here as they were in the preceding figures. Moreover, most of the fibers of the gracile fasciculus, which convey impulses originating in peripheral receptors stimulated by contact, pressure, and vibration in the lower part of the body, have terminated in the gracile nucleus (3) at this level. Axons of secondary neurons in the gracile nucleus emerge as internal arcuate fibers (13), which follow a semicircular course in the plane of the section, cross the midline, and accumulate as the medial lemniscus (10, Fig. 9), a prominent tract all the way to its termination in the thalamus (Figs. 9 to 27). Much of the cuneate fasciculus (20), which consists of primary fibers originating in the upper part of the body, is still present, but this fasciculus too, is being replaced by the cuneate nucleus (21) as the fibers of the fasciculus synapse in that nucleus.

Ventral to the cuneate nucleus and tract are the spinal trigeminal nucleus and tract (19 and 25). In the previous section, the spinal trigeminal tract was immediately beneath the pia mater. Here it is covered by the posterior spinocerebellar tract (24), which crosses the spinal trigeminal tract obliquely to reach the inferior cerebellar peduncle on the dorsal surface of the medulla (28, Fig. 10). When surgeons cut the spinal trigeminal tract for relief of intractable pain in the face, they necessarily also cut a part of the posterior spinocerebellar tract. This results in some impairment in the smooth, coordinated movements of the leg, thereby revealing something of the function of the posterior spinocerebellar tract. As this tract shifts to a dorsal position, the anterior spinocerebellar tract (33) moves into the relative position the posterior tract had occupied. Indeed, most of the tracts in the anterior aspect of the spinal cord, chiefly the

vestibulospinal (35) and anterior spinothalamic (38) tracts, are necessarily more laterally situated in the medulla, since the corticospinal fibers (118) which constitute the medullary pyramids occupy the anterior aspect of the medulla oblongata. Because a large group of corticospinal fibers is decussating, the left pyramid appears to slant dorsally and to the right in this figure.

The lower end of the hypoglossal nucleus (6) is only just included in the section. Lateral and ventral to it is a large, ill defined area, the reticular formation (34), bounded ventrally by the pyramids and dorsally by the trigeminal, gracile, and cuneate nuclei. Anatomically, it contains many nuclei widely dispersed in the white matter. As an anatomic region of varying size and boundaries it can be followed readily into the rostral mesencephalon (Fig. 24). Its neural connections mediate diverse functions. Reflex centers of vital functions, such as respiration and blood pressure, are resident in it, as are centers facilitating and inhibiting tonus of skeletal muscle. Other neurons in the reticular formation propagate impulses rostrally which affect the functional state of the thalamus and thereby the cerebral cortex. The anatomical basis of these several functions is not yet fully established. The vital segmental reflex centers receive impulses via collateral branches of primary fibers in several cranial nerves, but chiefly, the VIIth, IXth, and Xth. Collateral axons from many of the ascending and descending supra-segmental tracts synapse in other reticular nuclei which affect tonus, movement, and the functional state of the thalamus and cerebral cortex. The medial lemniscus, notably, does not.

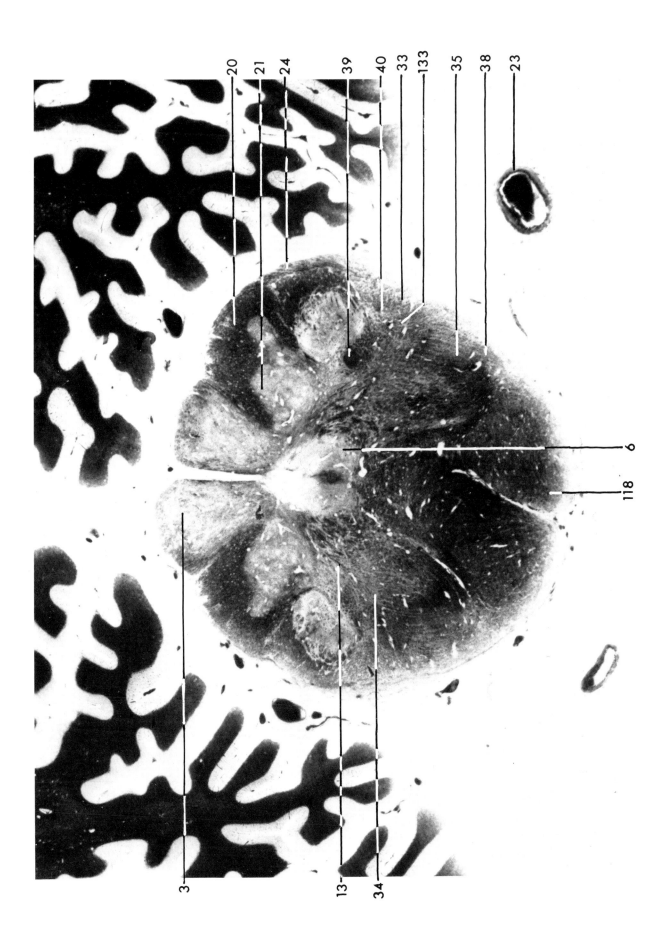

FIGURE 9.
Medulla Oblongata, Caudal Edge of the Inferior Olive

The dorsal part of the medulla resembles that of the preceding section, except that the accessory cuneate nucleus (44) is now present among the fibers of the cuneate fasciculus (20). This nucleus receives large myelinated axons of primary neurons of cervical nerves and is comparable to the dorsal nucleus in that it conveys to the cerebellum impulses initiated in receptors of the muscles, joints, (and tendons). To do this, secondary fibers emerge from the accessory cuneate nucleus, intermingle with the posterior spinocerebellar tract (24), and ascend into the cerebellum in the inferior cerebellar peduncle (28, Figs. 10 to 14 and 48 to 54). Both tracts facilitate the smooth and rapid execution of coordinated movements of the body and extremities by conveying impulses to the cerebellum from the muscles.

The internal arcuate fibers (13), which arise in the gracile (3) and cuneate (21) nuclei, extend in a semicircular course through the reticular formation, cross the midline, turn sharply, and ascend as a compact mass of fibers called the medial lemniscus (10). Fibers arising in the gracile nucleus cross first and accumulate progressively dorsal to the pyramid, followed by those from the cuneate nucleus which laminate dorsal to those already present in the medial lemniscus. Thus, impulses mediating tactile and position sense which are initiated in the leg are propagated upward in the anterior part of the medial lemniscus, with the foot being the most ventral; impulses from more rostral parts of the body and the arms are transmitted in progressively more dorsal fibers of the medial lemniscus. The medial lemniscus is the tract propagating nerve impulses originating in proprioceptive and tactile receptors in the muscles, tendons, joints, and skin toward conscious levels. Impulses initiated in these same receptors also reach the cerebellum, but chiefly via spinocerebellar tracts and the external arcuate fibers arising in the accessory cuneate nucleus (44), as already outlined. Only the medial lemniscus can properly be called a sensory tract, since one is never aware of impulses reaching the cerebellum.

There is no visible demarcation between the fibers of the medial lemniscus (10), the tectospinal tract (9), and the medial longitudinal fasciculus (8). No doubt there is considerable interdigitation. The medial longitudinal fasciculus, one of the long tracts in the brain stem (see 8, Fig. 39), is of varied composition. At the level of this section, most of the fibers are descending and have their origins chiefly in the medial vestibular nucleus (128, Figs. 11 to 14). Fibers continue into the spinal cord (8, Figs. 5 and 6). They effect reflex turning of the head and neck in response to vestibular stimulation. The tectospinal tract arises largely in the superior colliculus (210, Fig. 23) in the tectum of the mesencephalon, hence its name. The superior colliculus receives nerve fibers originating in the retina and fibers from the body, via the spinotectal tract. The tectospinal tract is the efferent outflow from the superior colliculus to the upper part of the spinal cord, completing suprasegmental reflexes initiated in the eye.

Several cranial nerve nuclei are present; the receptive spinal trigeminal nucleus (19) and motor hypoglossal nucleus (6) have already been noted in caudal figures. Dorsolateral to the hypoglossal nucleus is the dorsal motor nucleus of the vagus (17), the source of preganglionic fibers to thoracic and abdominal viscera. Vagal fibers to the skeletal muscles of branchiomeric origin arise in the ambiguus nucleus (32); it is too slender to be visible in Weigert sections. Hypoglossal and both vagal nuclei are nearly coextensive throughout the length of the medulla.

Lateral to the dorsal motor nucleus of the vagus (17) are the nucleus and tractus solitarius (18). The tract at this caudal level is made up of general visceral afferent axons whose cell bodies are located in the inferior ganglia of the vagus and glossopharyngeal nerves and in the geniculate ganglion of the facial nerve. These primary fibers enter the rostral medulla and caudal pons to form the slender descending solitary tract (Figs. 13 to 9) before they synapse in the equally slender solitary nucleus. The axons arising in this caudal part of the nucleus mediate reflexes or ascend to conscious levels in the thalamus, but by pathways which are not established. The caudal half of the solitary tract and the spinal trigeminal tract are similar; the first contains all the general visceral afferent fibers of cranial nerves VII, IX, and X. The spinal trigeminal tract contains general somatic afferent fibers of cranial nerves V, VII, IX, and X: the names conceal the varied composition of both tracts.

The medial (15) and inferior (16) olivary nuclei are just beginning to appear. More important is the lateral reticular nucleus (41). It probably receives impulses initiated in tactile receptors in the skin and conveys them to the cerebellum via the inferior cerebellar peduncle (28, Fig. 10). This pathway complements the spinocerebellar tracts and dorsal external arcuate fibers, which convey impulses initiated by receptors in the muscles, tendons, and joints. Thus, the cerebellum receives impulses initiated by both proprioceptive and exteroceptive receptors.

3—Gracile nucleus
8—Medial longitudinal fasciculus
9—Tectospinal tract
10—Medial lemniscus
13—Internal arcuate fibers
14—Pyramid
15—Medial accessory olivary nucleus
16—Inferior olivary nucleus
17—Dorsal nucleus of the vagus nerve
18—Nucleus and tractus solitarius
19—Spinal trigeminal nucleus
20—Cuneate fasciculus
21—Cuneate nucleus
24—Posterior spinocerebellar tract
25—Spinal tract of the trigeminal nerve
32—Ambiguus nucleus
33—Anterior spinocerebellar tract
39—Pick's bundle
40—Rubrospinal tract
41—Lateral reticular nucleus
44—Accessory cuneate nucleus

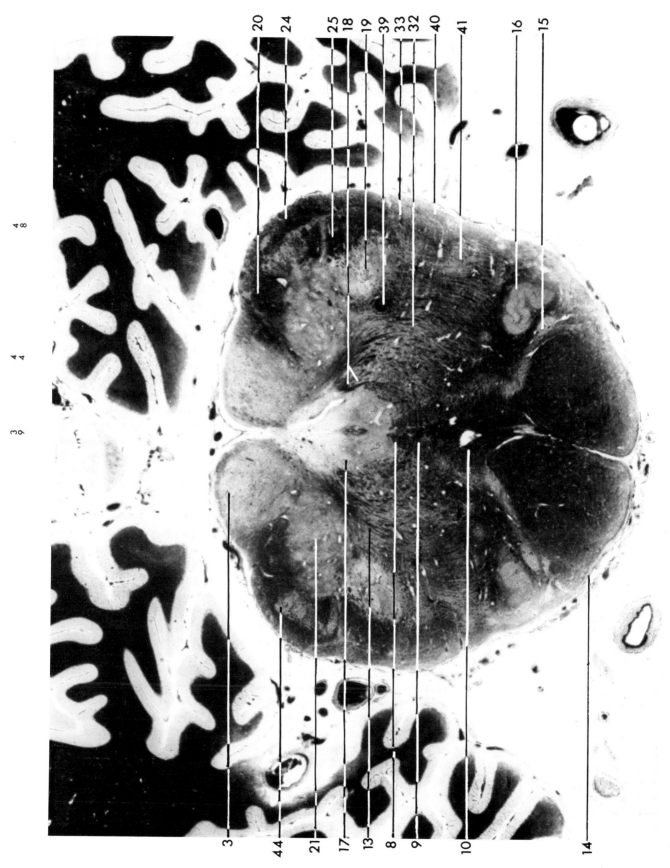

20
24
25
18
19
39
33
32
40
41
16
15

4
8

4
4

3
9

3
44
21
17
13
8
9
10
14

FIGURE 10.

Medulla Oblongata, Caudal Third of the Inferior Olive

Although the plane of section is now rostral to the gracile and cuneate nuclei, the accessory cuneate nucleus (44) is still present and the internal arcuate fibers still pursue a semicircular course through the reticular formation to enter the contralateral medial lemniscus (10), where they ascend to the posterolateral ventral nucleus of the thalamus (336, Fig. 27). The position of the gracile nucleus at lower levels is now occupied by the inferior vestibular nucleus (127). Axons from this nucleus ascend in the medial longitudinal fasciculus and terminate, in part, in the abducens (121, Fig. 15), trochlear (208, Fig. 21), and oculomotor (201, Fig. 23) nuclei. Movements of the head effect reflex adjustments of the eyes via such fibers from the inferior and the other vestibular nuclei. Two additional tracts may be mentioned here. The ventral central trigeminal tract (31) contains the secondary fibers arising from neurons in the spinal trigeminal nucleus which convey painful and thermal impulses originating in the face to conscious levels in the posteromedial ventral nucleus of the thalamus (332, Fig. 27). There is a variety of opinions but little concrete evidence as to the position of the tract. In this atlas it is placed tentatively between the inferior olive and the medial lemniscus (10). An alternative opinion places it close to the medial side of the lateral spinothalamic tract (133). It is homologous to the lateral spinothalamic tract.

Although the position of secondary fibers is largely unknown, pain in the face, which can be quite excruciating, has been effectively eliminated by surgical section of primary fibers in the spinal tract of the trigeminal nerve (25) at about this level; most of the posterior spinocerebellar fibers have already crossed the tract and entered the inferior cerebellar peduncle (28). Because these fibers are spared,

there is minimal impairment of coordination of movements, but the descending primary fibers mediating pain are cut before they have synapsed in the spinal trigeminal nucleus (19). This operation indicates that only the caudal part of the spinal trigeminal nucleus mediates painful stimuli arising in the face.

The dorsal longitudinal fasciculus (5) appears as a group of fibers dorsal to the hypoglossal nucleus (6). Some of these descending fibers may convey impulses from the hypothalamus, an important visceral reflex center, to the dorsal motor nucleus of the vagus (17), the chief source of preganglionic parasympathetic fibers.

The vertebral arteries (23), one of the two major sources of blood to the brain (the other being the internal carotid), are included here as well as in the preceding and following sections. The anterior spinal artery, which arises from the vertebral arteries, vascularizes a prismatic segment of the medulla including the hypoglossal nucleus (6) and nerve, medial longitudinal fasciculus (8), tectospinal tract (9), medial lemniscus (10), and corticospinal fibers (118) in the pyramids. Interruption of blood flow in the anterior spinal artery may result in a crossed paralysis. The ipsilateral side of the tongue is paralyzed because the hypoglossal nerve is directly involved, while the contralateral muscles of the body are also paralyzed, because the corticospinal fibers are injured above the level at which they cross (Fig. 8). In addition, there may be loss of a sense of position and of passive movements of the arm and leg on the side opposite to the damaged medial lemniscus (10). Unnamed branches of the vertebral arteries vascularize adjacent lateral wedges of the medulla, including the inferior olive and the reticular formation. Another branch of the vertebral artery is the posterior inferior cerebellar artery (30, Fig.

12), which supplies most of the rest of the medulla at this level, although the posterior spinal artery, which is also a vertebral branch, supplies some of the dorsal aspect of the medulla; it is a more important vessel further caudal in the medulla than here.

5—Dorsal longitudinal fasciculus
6—Hypoglossal nucleus
9—Tectospinal tract
10—Medial lemniscus
13—Internal arcuate fibers
15—Medial accessory olivary nucleus
17—Dorsal nucleus of the vagus nerve
18—Nucleus and tractus solitarius
23—Vertebral artery
28—Inferior cerebellar peduncle
31—Ventral central trigeminal tract
33—Anterior spinocerebellar tract
35—Vestibulospinal tract
39—Pick's bundle
40—Rubrospinal tract
41—Lateral reticular nucleus
44—Accessory cuneate nucleus
118—Corticospinal fibers
123—Central tegmental tract
127—Inferior vestibular nucleus
133—Lateral spinothalamic tract

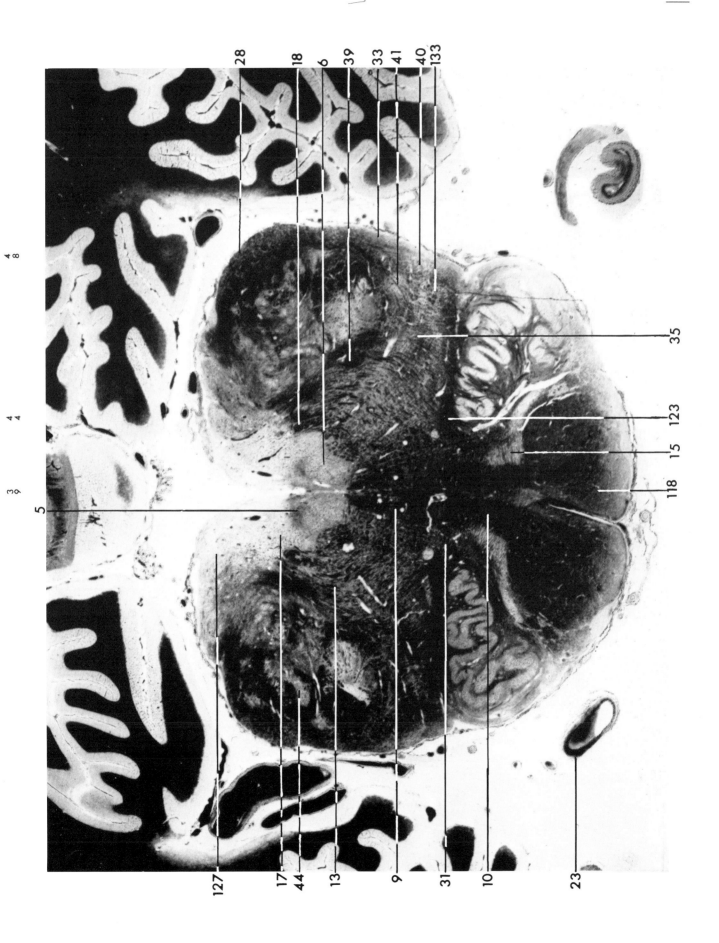

28 18 6 39 33 41 40 133

35

123

15

118

127 17 44 13 9 31 10 23

4 8

4 4

3 9

5

FIGURE 11.
Medulla Oblongata, Open Part of the Fourth Ventricle

This figure illustrates the caudal end of the so called open portion of the fourth ventricle (105). Since the thin posterior medullary velum (43) is usually torn in dissections, it was originally thought that the fourth ventricle was "open" to the subarachnoid space. However, thin though it is, the posterior medullary velum is sufficiently tough that it is not ruptured in hydrocephalus, even though the internal pressure of cerebrospinal fluid is enough seriously to compress brain tissue against the skull.

Since the medial vestibular nucleus (128) is one of the few structures not previously present at more caudal levels, a few comments about the VIIIth nerve are appropriate. Fibers of the vestibular division enter the brain stem at the juncture of the medulla and pons as one of the two components of the acoustic nerve (149, Fig. 14). Some of these primary fibers descend as small bundles, scattered within the inferior vestibular nucleus (127), to synapse in it and in the medial vestibular nucleus (128). If they had been grouped into one compact bundle, these special somatic afferent fibers would have been called a tract and given a name. "Inferior vestibular tract" or "spinal vestibular tract" would have been a logical name, since the fibers are comparable to the general somatic afferent fibers constituting the spinal trigeminal tract (25) and to the general and special visceral afferent fibers of the tractus solitarius (18). Fibers arising from neurons of the medial vestibular nucleus both ascend and descend in the medial longitudinal fasciculus (8). From about this level rostral into the mesencephalon this fasciculus contains fibers coursing in both directions. Caudal to this level the medial longitudinal fasciculus is chiefly, if not wholly, a descending tract. Fibers arising in the in-

ferior vestibular nucleus ascend in the medial longitudinal fasciculus to nuclei of the IIIrd, IVth, and VIth cranial nerves, as do those of the medial vestibular nucleus, but they do not descend. Both medial and inferior vestibular nuclei also have axons which reach the cerebellum via a subdivision of the inferior cerebellar peduncle (28) called the juxtarestiform body (139, Figs. 15, 48, and 49). All of these connections mediate reflex movements of the eyes and head.

The inferior cerebellar peduncle is just beginning to enlarge as more fibers accumulate in it. Olivocerebellar fibers should now be added to those already mentioned (dorsal spinocerebellar, dorsal external arcuate, and reticulocerebellar from the lateral reticular nucleus). Most of the very numerous olivocerebellar fibers arise in the inferior olive (16) contralateral of the peduncle, course through both medial lemnisci (10) and the opposite inferior olive, to enter the reticular formation, where they are visible here (27), before penetrating the spinal trigeminal tract and nucleus to reach the inferior cerebellar peduncle. The course of olivocerebellar fibers are more obvious in Figure 12.

Many impulses reach the inferior olive through the central tegmental tract (123) and are there transmitted to the olivocerebellar tract. The central tegmental tract, which can be followed as a distinct bundle from the rostral mesencephalon (Fig. 24), is actually a composite bundle of both ascending and descending fibers. Descending fibers to the inferior olive arise in the rostral part of the red nucleus (214, Figs. 27 to 29) and in the reticular formation in the tegmentum of the mesencephalon (Figs. 23 to 21). Thus the cerebellum receives impulses not only from the periphery of the body but from centers higher in the brain as

well, including the cerebral hemispheres, via this central tegmental tract and the olivocerebellar pathway.

5—Dorsal longitudinal fasciculus
8—Medial longitudinal fasciculus
14—Pyramid
16—Inferior olivary nucleus
17—Dorsal nucleus of the vagus nerve
18—Nucleus and tractus solitarius
19—Spinal trigeminal nucleus
25—Spinal tract of the trigeminal nerve
27—Olivocerebellar tract
31—Ventral central trigeminal tract
32—Ambiguus nucleus
33—Anterior spinocerebellar tract
39—Pick's bundle
40—Rubrospinal tract
43—Posterior medullary velum
105—Fourth ventricle
123—Central tegmental tract
127—Inferior vestibular nucleus
128—Medial vestibular nucleus

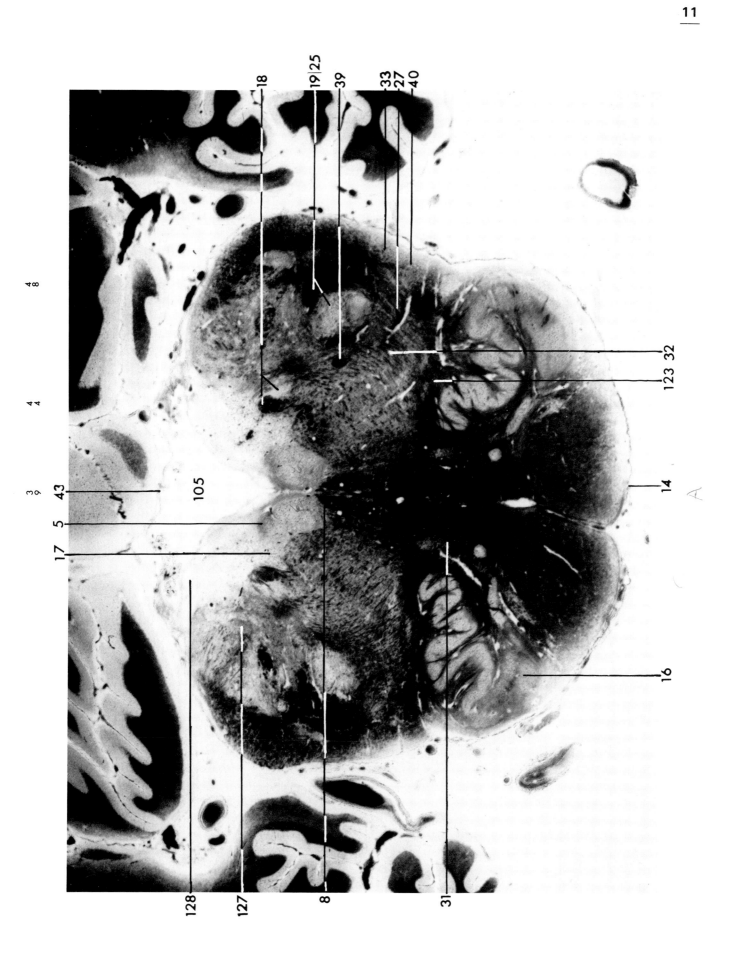

FIGURE 12. Medulla Oblongata, Midsection

A midmedullary level is usually selected for demonstrating the orderly array of the cell columns related to the cranial nerves. Most medial is the somatic motor column, here represented by the hypoglossal nucleus (6). Root fibers of the hypoglossal nerve are visible just lateral to the medial longitudinal fasciculus (8) and tectospinal tract (9), and can be traced toward their emergence between the pyramids (14) and the inferior olive (16). Immediately lateral to the hypoglossal nucleus, the dorsal motor nucleus of the vagus (17) represents the general visceral efferent column. The ambiguus nucleus (32), which symbolizes the special visceral motor column, has migrated from its primitive position to approach its principal source of impulses, the spinal trigeminal nucleus and tract (19 and 25). Thus the axons issuing from the ambiguus nucleus follow a recurrent course. They extend dorsomedially toward the hypoglossal and the dorsal motor nuclei but, before reaching these nuclei, the ambiguus fibers make a sharp turn to become recurrent and emerge from the brain stem midway between the inferior olive (16) and the inferior cerebellar peduncle (28). It is suggested that the ambiguus nucleus may originally have occupied a position between the hypoglossal and dorsal motor nuclei, but since all special visceral motor nuclei save one have migrated, the primitive position between the somatic and general visceral motor nuclei is speculative.

Immediately lateral to the dorsal motor nucleus of the vagus are the nucleus and tractus solitarius (18). The tract contains primary afferent fibers that synapse upon the neurons of the solitary nucleus, which give rise to secondary fibers. Included in the tract are the central processes of both primary general visceral afferent (pain) and special visceral afferent (taste) fibers, which distribute themselves peripherally in the cranial nerves VII, IX, and X. Most taste fibers are contained in the glossopharyngeal nerve, and fewer in the facial nerve; the vagus includes a few from the anterior surface of the epiglottis. General visceral afferent fibers descend and synapse in the caudal part of the solitary nucleus. Taste fibers terminate in the more rostral part of the nucleus. At the level of this figure, taste fibers are probably ending in the nucleus. Thus the medulla contains four descending groups of primary fibers of cranial nerves: general somatic afferent (spinal trigeminal tract), general and special visceral afferent (solitary tract), and special somatic afferent (unnamed fibers) that occur in small clusters within the inferior vestibular nucleus (127) ventral of the leader.

This section also demonstrates how the symptoms of a common vascular lesion, such as the posterior inferior cerebellar artery (30) syndrome, can be related to the fiber tracts and nuclei resident in the region of the lesion. Loss of pain and temperature sensibility on the opposite side of the body results from damage to the lateral spinothalamic tract (133). These secondary fibers arise on the opposite side of the body and cross in the anterior white commissure of the spinal cord. Loss of pain and temperature sensibility and of reflex activity ipsilaterally in the face results from vascular impairment affecting the primary and hence uncrossed fibers of the spinal trigeminal tract (25). This tract is now obscured by olivocerebellar fibers coursing toward the inferior cerebellar peduncle (28), but the spinal trigeminal nucleus (19) is quite visible. Speech also is affected, and examination shows paralysis of a vocal cord and the soft palate, since the ambiguus nucleus (32) and the motor fibers of the vagus arising therein are injured. Dizziness and conjugate eye movements to the side of the lesion may occur to varying degrees if there is irritation of the inferior and medial vestibular nuclei (127 and 128). Impairment of blood supply to the anterior spinocerebellar tract (33) and the posterior spinocerebellar tract now in the inferior cerebellar peduncle (28) would produce incoordination of the arm and leg on the side of the vascular injury, compounded by the degree to which the cerebellum itself was deprived of blood. Injury of fibers in the reticular formation that descend to the intermediolateral cell column (N, Fig. 5) of the upper thoracic cord also may result in a drooping of the ipsilateral eyelid and constriction of the pupil (Horner's syndrome).

Olivocerebellar fibers (27) are only labeled in the medial olivary nucleus, but they can be seen traversing both medial lemnisci, the contralateral inferior olive, and the spinal trigeminal tract into the inferior cerebellar peduncle (28).

6—Hypoglossal nucleus
9—Tectospinal tract
10—Medial lemniscus
17—Dorsal nucleus of the vagus nerve
18—Nucleus and tractus solitarius
23—Vertebral artery
27—Olivocerebellar tract
28—Inferior cerebellar peduncle (restiform body)
29—Dorsal accessory olivary nucleus
30—Posterior inferior cerebellar artery
31—Ventral central trigeminal tract
33—Anterior spinocerebellar tract
34—Reticular formation
35—Vestibulospinal tract
40—Rubrospinal tract
118—Corticospinal fibers
127—Inferior vestibular nucleus
128—Medial vestibular nucleus
133—Lateral spinothalamic tract

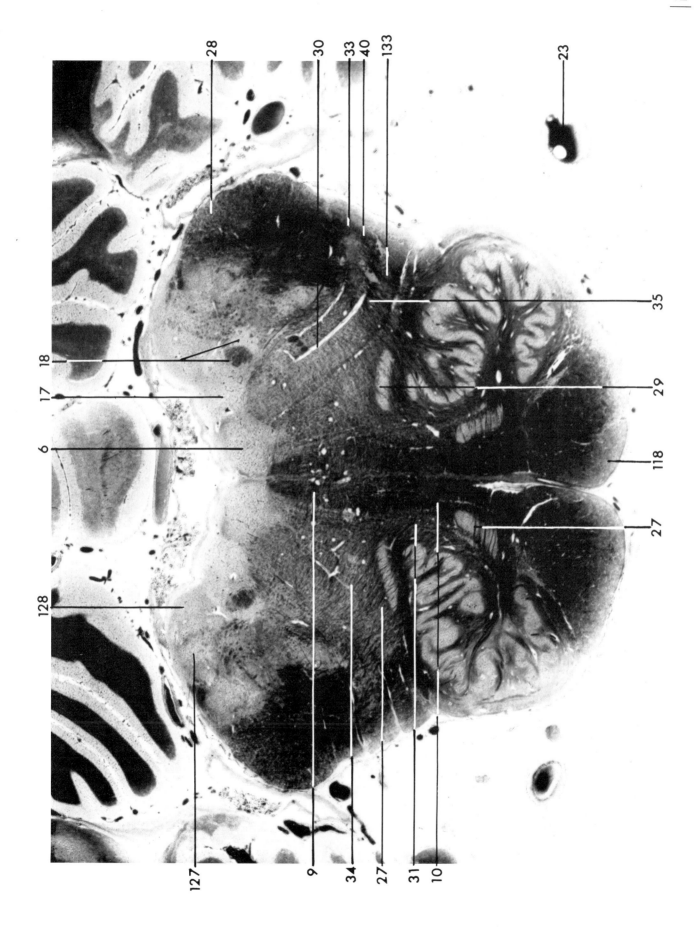

FIGURE 13. Rostral End of the Medulla Oblongata

Figure 13 is close to the junction of the medulla with the pons. Therefore, the two lateral spaces posterior of the dorsal cochlear nuclei (144) are the lateral foramina (147), which connect the fourth ventricle and the subarachnoid space. The tela choroidea (12) is labeled in the roof of the fourth ventricle (105) and again where it extends through the lateral foramina into the subarachnoid space. A minor amount of cerebrospinal fluid is thus secreted directly into this subarachnoid space. Most cerebrospinal fluid is secreted internally by the tela choroidea of the lateral (408, Figs. 22 to 38), third (311, Figs. 27 to 31), and fourth ventricles and flows through these lateral foramina and a medial foramen into the subarachnoid space.

The dorsal cochlear nucleus (144) is adherent to the dorsal surface of the inferior cerebellar peduncle, which has become massive because so many olivocerebellar fibers are now contained in it. However, additional olivocerebellar fibers (27) still extend through the reticular formation, spinal trigeminal nucleus, and tract (19, 25), obscuring them, to enter the peduncle. The many small bundles of primary myelinated fibers descending in the inferior vestibular nucleus (127) give it a speckled appearance. This nucleus might have been labeled the lateral vestibular nucleus (143), as it is in the next section, since there is no visible indication of transition from one nucleus to the other in Weigert sections. The lateral vestibular nucleus is said to be present at the level of entrance of the acoustic nerve and to extend rostrally. The inferior vestibular nucleus extends caudally from the entrance of the nerve. This figure includes the glossopharyngeal nerve (42).

The nucleus and tractus solitarius (18) are small here, since the figure is so close to the level of entrance of the facial nerve, which is the most rostral of the cranial nerves that contribute to the tract. Although the glossopharyngeal nerve (42) contains most of the fibers

mediating taste, not many have entered the tract at this level.

The area of the reticular formation is considerable. This region is bounded by the vestibular nuclei dorsally, by the inferior cerebellar peduncle (28), lateral spinothalamic tract (133) and the anterior spinocerebellar tract (33) laterally, and inferior olive (16) ventrally; the medial longitudinal fasciculus and tectospinal tract are medial. It contains important reflex centers mediating vital functions of respiration and blood pressure. As previously mentioned, many ascending suprasegmental tracts, but not the medial lemniscus (10). give off collateral branches into regional reticular nuclei and propagate impulses into what is called the ascending reticular activating system, which affects the functioning of the thalami and, through them, the cerebral hemispheres. Reticulospinal tracts (K, Figs. 1 to 6), which have a major effect upon the tonus of skeletal muscles, arise from still other neurons in the reticular formation. Apparently most of the fibers which inhibit tone originate in nuclei chiefly confined to the medulla oblongata, whereas facilitating reticulospinal fibers arise in pontine and mesencephalic as well as in medullary nuclei. The structural basis in the reticular formation of these various functions is still little known.

8—Medial longitudinal fasciculus
12—Tela choroidea of the fourth ventricle
14—Pyramid
16—Inferior olivary nucleus
18—Nucleus and tractus solitarius
19—Spinal trigeminal nucleus
25—Spinal tract of the trigeminal nerve
27—Olivocerebellar tract
31—Ventral central trigeminal tract
32—Ambiguus nucleus
33—Anterior spinocerebellar tract
40—Rubrospinal tract
42—Glossopharyngeal nerve
105—Fourth ventricle
123—Central tegmental tract
127—Inferior vestibular nucleus
128—Medial vestibular nucleus
144—Dorsal cochlear nucleus
147—Lateral foramen of Luschka

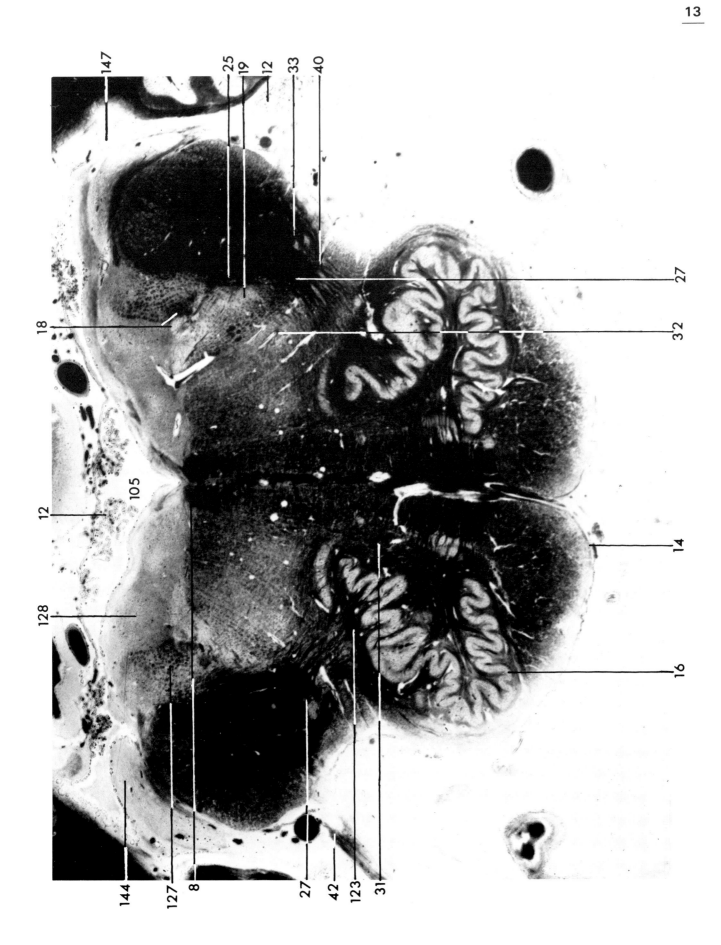

FIGURE 14. Junction of the Medulla Oblongata and Pons TRANSVERSE

Figure 14 provides an occasion for reviewing the components of the eighth nerve. The primary vestibular fibers of the acoustic nerve (149) enter ventral to the inferior cerebellar peduncle; most of them terminate in the lateral (143), superior (135), medial (128), and inferior vestibular nuclei, but some proceed directly to the cerebellum itself via the inferior cerebellar peduncle (28). Axons of secondary neurons in the medial and inferior vestibular nuclei (127, Fig. 13) also ascend into the cerebellum via the juxtarestiform body (139, Fig. 15) which is a subdivision of the inferior cerebellar peduncle. Another group of secondary fibers from all vestibular nuclei ascends in the medial longitudinal fasciculus to reach the abducens (121, Fig. 15), trochlear (208, Fig. 22), and oculomotor (201, Fig. 23) nuclei. Impulses traversing these fibers bring about the reflex movements of the eyes in response to stimuli arising in the vestibule and semicircular canals of the inner ear. Descending secondary fibers in the medial longitudinal fasciculus from the medial vestibular nucleus enter the cord in the medial longitudinal fasciculus (8, Figs. 5 and 6) to effect the reflex turning of the head. Although the lateral vestibular nucleus contributes some fibers to this tract, its major outflow is the vestibulospinal tract (35), which can be followed from Figure 12 caudally to the sacral spinal cord, Figure 1. The vestibulospinal tract terminates chiefly upon interneurons of the anterior gray horn; its impulses tend to increase tonus in extensor muscles. Although impulses initiated in the vestibular nerve do not reach consciousness, the path is not known, and there is no English word for this special sensibility, as there are for sight and sound. One is aware of vestibular impulses primarily when they conflict with other sensory impressions, as in dizziness.

The primary fibers in the auditory division of the acoustic nerve (149) arise in the cochlea and terminate in the dorsal (144, Fig. 13) and ventral cochlear (148) nuclei on the dorsal and lateral surfaces of the inferior cerebellar peduncle (28). The sensory path toward the thalamus from these two nuclei takes an oblique course rostrally, with several intermediate synapses, so that its decussation in the trapezoid body (101) does not occur until the level of Figure 17. Rostral to the decussation, the auditory tract continues laterally, still on an oblique course, then turns directly rostral as a prominent tract, now called the lateral lemniscus (136, Fig. 18) to reach the inferior colliculus (209, Fig. 20), on its way to the medial geniculate nucleus (333, Fig. 23). A few fibers bypass a synapse in this nucleus and directly enter the brachium of the inferior colliculus (222, Fig. 21) to terminate in the medial geniculate body.

The inferior cerebellar peduncle (28) is labeled several times because the tract makes a sharp turn dorsally, which is visible within the plane of this section, to enter the cerebellum. Throughout the length of the medulla the fibers are oriented in the rostral-caudal direction, and it is just beyond the entrance of the eighth nerve that the peduncle makes this sharp change in direction, as if it had been held down by the embrace of the dorsal auditory division and the ventral vestibular division of the acoustic nerve. Fibers of the peduncle are at first a compact mass in the white matter of the cerebellum as they arch over the dorsal surface of the dentate nucleus (137).

The deep nuclei of the cerebellum (fastigial (120), globose (126), emboliform (130), dentate (137)) extend across the top of the figure. These nuclei give rise to most of the efferent fibers that leave the cerebellum via the superior (211) and inferior (28) cerebellar peduncles. (The middle cerebellar peduncle (142) is a purely afferent tract.) The deep nuclei receive impulses from the cerebellar cortex via axons of Purkinje cells and by collateral branches from some, if not all, afferent fibers to the cerebellar cortex in the superior, middle, and inferior peduncles.

Efferent fibers arise in both the ipsi- and contralateral fastigial nuclei. These are fastigiovestibular fibers to all four vestibular nuclei and fastigioreticular to the reticular nuclei. They traverse the juxtarestiform body (139, Fig. 15). By way of efferent fibers from these vestibular and reticular nuclei, which were earlier identified, the cerebellum indirectly influences the activity of spinal motor neurons innervating skeletal muscle.

In addition, efferent fibers that originate in globose, emboliform, and dentate nuclei collect to form the superior cerebellar peduncle (211). This peduncle can be followed rostrally in the following sections through its decussation (200, Fig. 21) to terminations in the contralateral red nucleus (214, Fig. 25) and some thalamic nuclei that in part have efferent connections to the cerebral cortex. These are chiefly the intermediate ventral (337, Fig. 30), anterior ventral (329, Fig. 36), and small intralaminar nuclei in the internal medullary lamina (339, Figs. 28 to 34). Some fibers also descend to nuclei in the brain stem. Through these several fiber tracts, the cerebellum is able to modulate neural activity of cerebral cortical neurons (red nucleus and thalamus) and spinal motor neurons (vestibular and reticular nuclei). In turn, the cerebellum is affected by impulses propagated in cerebral, reticular, and vestibular neurons. The vestibular pathways are described in the first paragraph. The major cortical pathway via corticopontine and pontocerebellar fibers will be introduced as they appear in the figures.

The two vertebral arteries (23) are sectioned obliquely as they converge to unite and form the basilar artery (102, Fig. 18).

9—Tectospinal tract
10—Medial lemniscus
23—Vertebral artery
27—Olivocerebellar tract
28—Inferior cerebellar peduncle
31—Ventral central trigeminal tract
33—Anterior spinocerebellar tract
40—Rubrospinal tract
43—Posterior medullary velum
105—Fourth ventricle
118—Corticospinal fibers
120—Fastigial nucleus
123—Central tegmental tract
126—Globose nucleus
128—Medial vestibular nucleus
130—Emboliform nucleus
133—Lateral spinothalamic tract
135—Superior vestibular nucleus
137—Dentate nucleus
142—Middle cerebellar peduncle
143—Lateral vestibular nucleus
148—Ventral cochlear nucleus
149—Acoustic nerve
211—Superior cerebellar peduncle

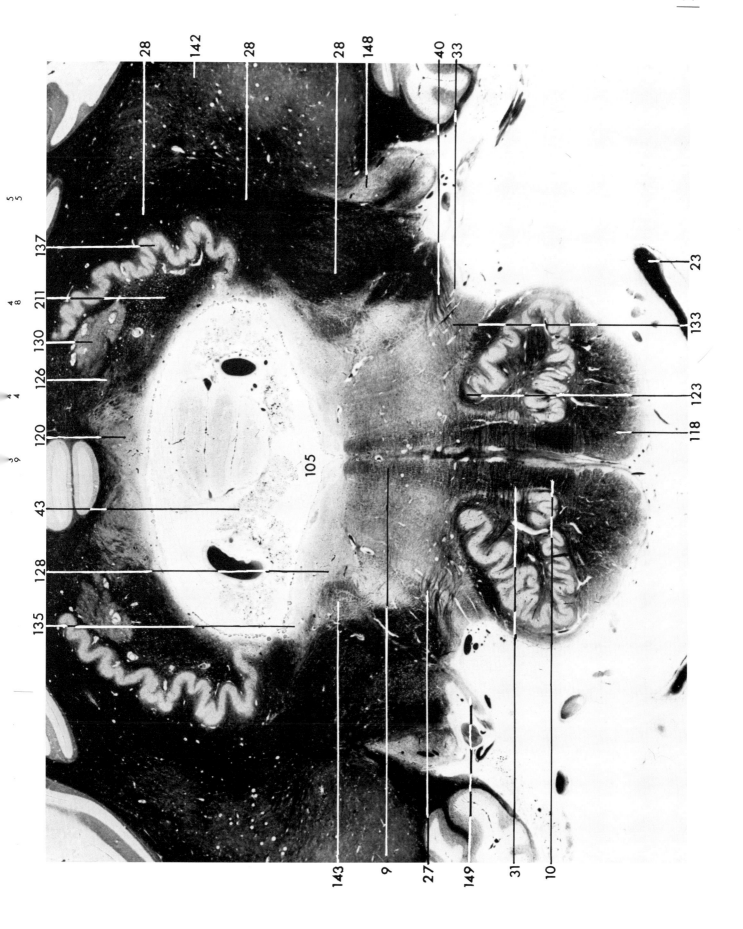

FIGURE 15. Caudal Edge of the Pons

The configuration of the brain stem changes sharply at the junction of the pons and medulla. The medial lemnisci (10), which are tall slender columns in the medulla, are here compact oval masses, and in following sections will spread out into masses which are flat in the horizontal plane. It is as though the inferior olives (16), of which only the rostral tip of one is still visible, had supported the lemnisci upright. The medial longitudinal fasciculus (8) and tectospinal tract (9), however, remain close to the midline in the floor of the fourth ventricle. Corticospinal tracts still resemble the medullary pyramids, but they are now covered ventrally by pontocerebellar fibers (103). The central tegmental tracts (123) have become compact masses whose relation to the inferior olives is obvious in parasagittal section (Fig. 45). Rubro-olivary fibers are a major component of the tract.

The elevation in the floor of the fourth ventricle (105) caused in part by the somatic motor abducens nucleus (121) is the facial colliculus. The spinal trigeminal nucleus and tract (19 and 25) are no longer obscured by the olivocerebellar fibers. Ventral and medial to these trigeminal components is the facial nucleus (131), which gives origin to fibers supplying the branchiomeric muscles of facial expression.

The superior olivary nucleus (132) ventral to the facial nucleus (131) can serve to represent a number of nuclei involved in the conduction of impulses to consciousness initiated in the cochlea. The auditory pathway departs from the pattern typical of most other sensory systems, in which a primary and secondary neuron conduct nerve impulses from the peripheral receptor to the thalamus. (This enumeration always omits small internuncial neurons between the primary and the secondary neuron.) In the atypical auditory pathway, there is a series of relay nuclei, such as the superior olive, the nuclei of the lateral lemniscus (151, Fig. 18) and trapezoid body, and the inferior colliculus (209, Fig. 19), which are interposed between the dorsal and ventral cochlear nuclei and the medial geniculate nucleus (333, Fig. 23). Because these nuclei are interconnected across the midline, a lesion in the auditory system does not result in unilateral deafness unless the lesion involves the ear itself or the acoustic nerve.

Figure 15 shows all three of the cerebellar peduncles, the inferior (28), the superior (211), in the lateral part of the anterior medullary velum (119), and the middle (142). The inferior peduncle, as already reviewed, is primarily an afferent tract, but it contains also the efferent fastigioreticular and fastigiovestibular fibers, which enter the brain stem via the juxtarestiform body (139) in the medial edge of the inferior cerebellar peduncle. Similarly, while the superior peduncle is primarily an efferent bundle, the anterior spinocerebellar tract (33) is the best known of the afferent fibers it contains. Nerve impulses course rostrally in the tract where it is labeled in the ventral lateral edge of the tegmentum of the pons. In Figure 16 the tract turns dorsally, crosses the efferent fibers of the superior peduncle, becomes incorporated in its medial edge, and, proceeding caudally, re-enters the present figure where the anterior spinocerebellar tract is labeled again in the superior cerebellar peduncle on its way to the cerebellum. Other afferent fibers in the superior peduncle arise in the mesencephalic nucleus of the trigeminal nerve and possibly in the superior and inferior colliculi. The middle cerebellar peduncle (142) is constituted entirely of afferent pontocerebellar fibers (103).

8—Medial longitudinal fasciculus
10—Medial lemniscus
16—Inferior olivary nucleus
19—Spinal trigeminal nucleus
23—Vertebral artery
25—Spinal trigeminal tract
28—Inferior cerebellar peduncle
31—Ventral central trigeminal tract
33—Anterior spinocerebellar tract
40—Rubrospinal tract
103—Pontocerebellar fibers
119—Anterior medullary velum
121—Abducens nucleus
123—Central tegmental tract
131—Facial nucleus
132—Superior olivary nucleus
133—Lateral spinothalamic tract
135—Superior vestibular nucleus
139—Juxtarestiform body
150—Trigeminal nerve
211—Superior cerebellar peduncle

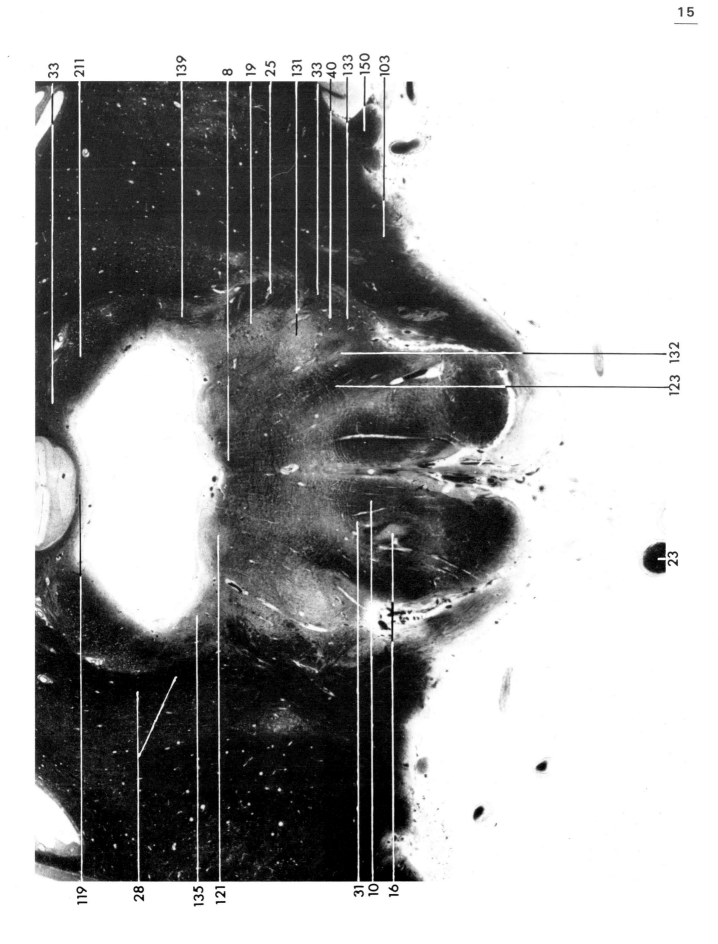

FIGURE 16. Level of the Facial Colliculus in the Pons

Although it is close to the previous section, Figure 16 is included because it is one of the major representative levels in the brain stem.

The major structure of the level is the facial nucleus (131). This nucleus, in the course of evolution, is thought to have migrated toward the source of its major stimulation, as have other branchiomeric motor nuclei. Its chief source of impulses is, of course, the spinal trigeminal nucleus (19), which propagates the impulses initiated by pain and temperature in the face. Because of this migration the efferent fibers of the facial nerve follow a recurrent course, much as do those of the ambiguus nucleus. The axons issue from the facial nucleus as numerous fibers, not distinct in the section, and course toward the abducens nucleus (121). Upon approaching the medial side of that nucleus, where the facial fibers are labeled (134), they turn rostrally and curve around the rostral aspect of the abducens nucleus and reappear in this section as a long compact group of fibers, obliquely oriented (134). It is not possible to follow them in this figure to their emergence from the brain stem at the caudal border of the pons, because it is just caudal to Figure 15. Medial to the facial fibers, the root fibers of the abducens nerve (146) also are directed inferiorly toward their emergence at the caudal border of the pons, and are labeled at several places in the tegmental and basilar portions of the pons. A lesion in the region where abducens and corticospinal (118) fibers are in proximity would result in a crossed paralysis: the body would be paralyzed on the side opposite the lesion, since the affected corticospinal fibers cross in the decussation of the pyramids (Fig. 8). Together with this contralateral bodily paralysis, the lateral rectus muscle of the ipsilateral eye would be paralyzed. That eye would not move laterally past the midline and, at rest, would be directed medially because of the muscular imbalance created.

The other component fibers of the facial nerve cannot be distinguished in the section although they are, of course, present. The parasympathetic, preganglionic fibers, which affect secretory activity in the glands of the nose and palate and in the lacrimal gland, have cell bodies in the superior salivatory nucleus. Its location is not known, although by analogy with the position of other general visceral efferent nuclei one would expect it to be somewhere between the somatic motor abducens nucleus, and the spinal trigeminal (19) and superior vestibular (135) nuclei. The few pain fibers of the facial nerve (general somatic afferent) which arise peripherally in the region of the external ear are incorporated in the spinal trigeminal tract (25). General visceral afferent fibers from the soft palate and palatine tonsil and taste fibers (special visceral afferent) are components of the tractus solitarius and synapse in its nucleus; the tract and nucleus become visible only at lower levels of the brain stem (18, Fig. 13).

This is the level of the brain stem at which the anterior spinocerebellar tract (33) curves dorsally, arches over, and enters the medial edge of the superior cerebellar peduncle, as discussed in connection with Figure 15. Most of the other comment there is also applicable here, as the two sections are close together.

Pontocerebellar fibers (103) are arbitrarily subdivided into two parts by the root fibers of the trigeminal nerve (150) in the pons. Medial to the nerve these fibers occupy the basilar portion of the pons, as do corticospinal fibers (118); lateral to the trigeminal nerve, the pontocerebellar fibers are usually called the middle cerebellar peduncle (142).

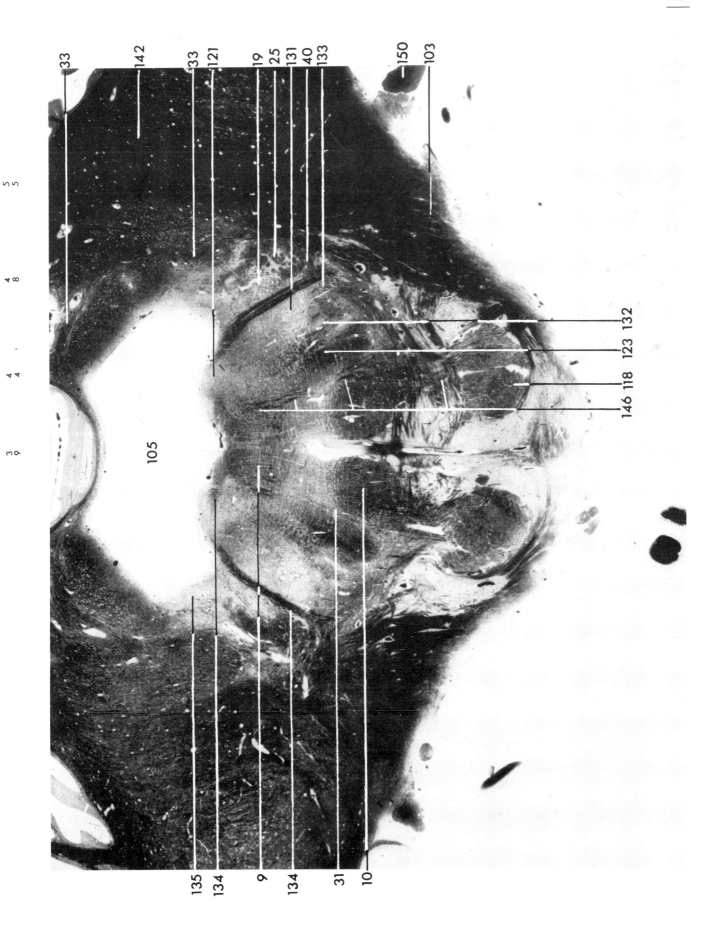

FIGURE 17.

Midpons and the Superior Sensory Trigeminal Nucleus

The level of the superior sensory (141) and motor (140) nuclei of the trigeminal nerve (150) is still another of the major levels of the brain stem. Those entering primary fibers which mediate pain and temperature in the face descend through inferior levels of the brain stem, as the spinal trigeminal tract (25), into the uppermost cervical spinal cord (B, Fig. 6) and synapse in the caudal one-third of the spinal trigeminal nucleus (19, Figs. 11 to 7). Other afferent fibers in the root of the trigeminal nerve (138), which convey impulses initiated in all varieties of tactile receptors, pass dorsomedially and synapse in the superior sensory nucleus of the trigeminal nerve (141) and also in the uppermost end of the spinal trigeminal nucleus. The motor nucleus of the trigeminal nerve (140) is medial to the superior sensory nucleus and is separated from it by the trigeminal root fibers (138). It is the only branchiomeric motor nucleus which has not migrated because, from the first, it has been adjacent to its major afferent input. Some trigeminal root fibers extend dorsally beyond these two nuclei as the mesencephalic tract of the trigeminal nerve (129). This tract consists of processes of primary neurons whose cell bodies are scattered along the tract; the tract extends into the rostral mesencephalon, but is visible only as far as Figure 19 in these figures. The mesencephalic nucleus is a notable exception to the rule that cell bodies of primary afferent fibers are located in ganglia outside the central nervous system. The mesencephalic nucleus and tract mediate position sensibility in the muscles of mastication and, possibly, in the extrinsic ocular muscles. The course and termination of its central processes (axons) are not known, although obviously impulses reach conscious levels.

The corticospinal (118) fibers are still compact masses resembling the medullary pyra-

mids, but are now buried in pontine nuclei (104) and pontocerebellar fibers (103). The pontocerebellar fibers arise from neurons in the pontine nuclei, cross the midline, and ascend into the cerebellum in the middle cerebellar peduncle (142). Pontine nuclei receive impulses from the cerebral cortex via corticopontine fibers. The large influx of neural information from the cerebrum, together with that coming from the periphery of the body via the several fiber tracts in the inferior and superior cerebellar peduncles, is integrated in the cerebellum; neural impulses resulting from this integration are emitted over fiber tracts in the superior and inferior peduncles, already described, and modulate neural activity in the cerebrum and brain stem.

Immediately dorsal to the basilar portion of the pons in the ventral part of the tegmentum are the medial lemnisci, which are now flattened into two masses whose fibers are cut transversely. The fibers that convey impulses initiated in peripheral receptors in the foot are localized most laterally in the opposite medial lemniscus, while those from progressively more rostral dermatomes are more and more medial in the medial lemniscus. The ventral central trigeminal tract (31) is tentatively placed in the dorsal edge of the medial lemniscus.

A single basilar artery (102) has now been formed by the union of the vertebral arteries. The long and short circumferential branches, named and unnamed, which arise from it vascularize most of the pons and cerebellum, and the occipital lobe of the cerebrum.

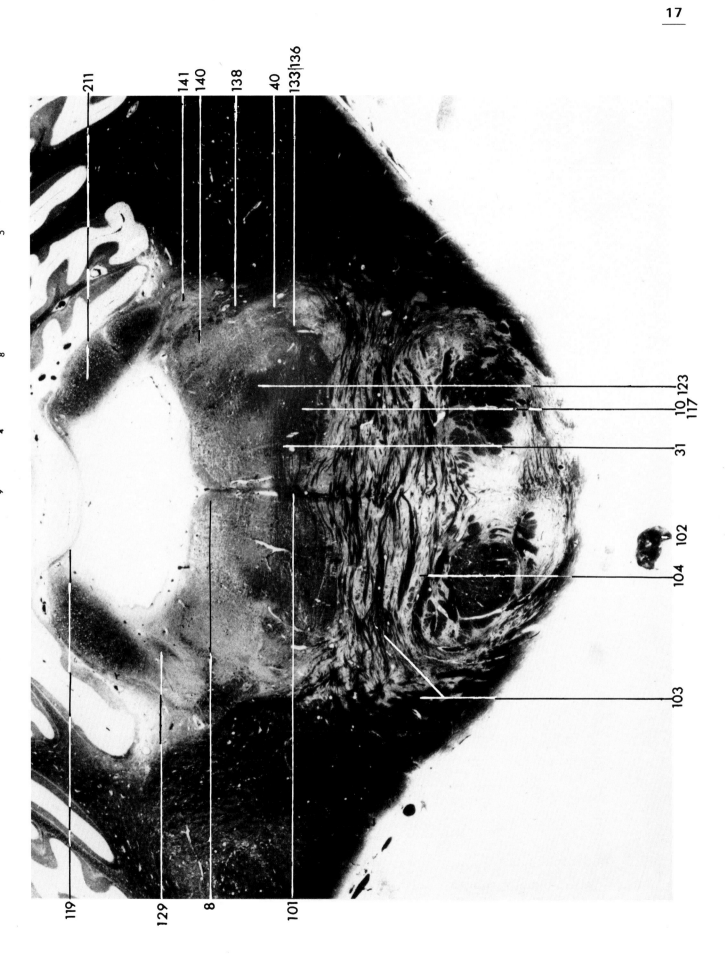

FIGURE 18. Rostral Pons

There are two major groups of fibers in the basilar portion of the pons. Corticopontine fibers (124) arise in all four lobes of the cerebral cortex, pass through the internal capsule (Figs. 38 to 27), and the crus cerebri (220, Figs. 30 to 21) to enter the basilar portion of the pons and synapse in the pontine nuclei (104). Pontocerebellar fibers (103) arise in the pontine nuclei, cross to the opposite side, and converge to form the middle cerebellar peduncle (142). Through this two-neuron pathway, the cerebellum receives impulses from the cerebral cortex which modulate the impulses emitted in turn from the cerebellum. Integrated impulses return to the cerebrum via the superior cerebellar peduncle (211) or reach nuclei in the brain stem via the juxtarestiform body (139, Fig. 15).

The second functional group of fibers includes the corticospinal (118) and corticobulbar (152) fibers. Corticobulbar fibers, like corticospinal fibers, arise in the cerebral cortex and traverse the internal capsule and crus cerebri, but terminate via a small internuncial neuron in those cranial nerve nuclei that effect volitional movements.

In the tegmentum of the pons the medial lemniscus (10) is now a flat fiber mass which is continuous laterally with the lateral spinothalamic tract (133), which mediates pain and temperature from the body, and with the lateral lemniscus (136), which mediates sound. The nucleus of the lateral lemniscus (151) is another of the relay nuclei in the auditory pathway, comparable with the superior olivary nucleus and the nucleus of the trapezoid body. The ventral central trigeminal tract (31), mediating pain and temperature sensations from the face, may be located in the dorsal part of the medial lemniscus, but this is largely conjecture. The course of the axons of secondary neurons which convey impulses originating in tactile and pressure receptors of the face to the posteromedial ventral thalamic nucleus

(332, Fig. 27) also is not well documented. These axons do arise in the superior sensory nucleus (141, Fig. 17) and possibly in the rostral end of the spinal trigeminal nucleus. As both crossed and direct fibers, they form a dorsal central trigeminal tract that is said to be located in the floor of the fourth ventricle (105), roughly ventral to the mesencephalic tract and nucleus of the trigeminal nerve (129).

The reticular formation is now appreciably reduced to the lightly myelinated area between the superior cerebellar peduncle (211), medial longitudinal fasciculus, and the medial lemniscus (10); it surrounds the central tegmental tract (123), which is the major tract of ascending and descending fibers of the reticular formation.

9—Tectospinal tract
10—Medial lemniscus
31—Ventral central trigeminal tract
40—Rubrospinal tract
102—Basilar artery
105—Fourth ventricle
118—Corticospinal fibers
123—Central tegmental tract
124—Corticopontine fibers
129—Mesencephalic nucleus and tract of the trigeminal nerve
133—Lateral spinothalamic tract
136—Lateral lemniscus
142—Middle cerebellar peduncle
151—Nucleus of the lateral lemniscus
152—Corticobulbar fibers

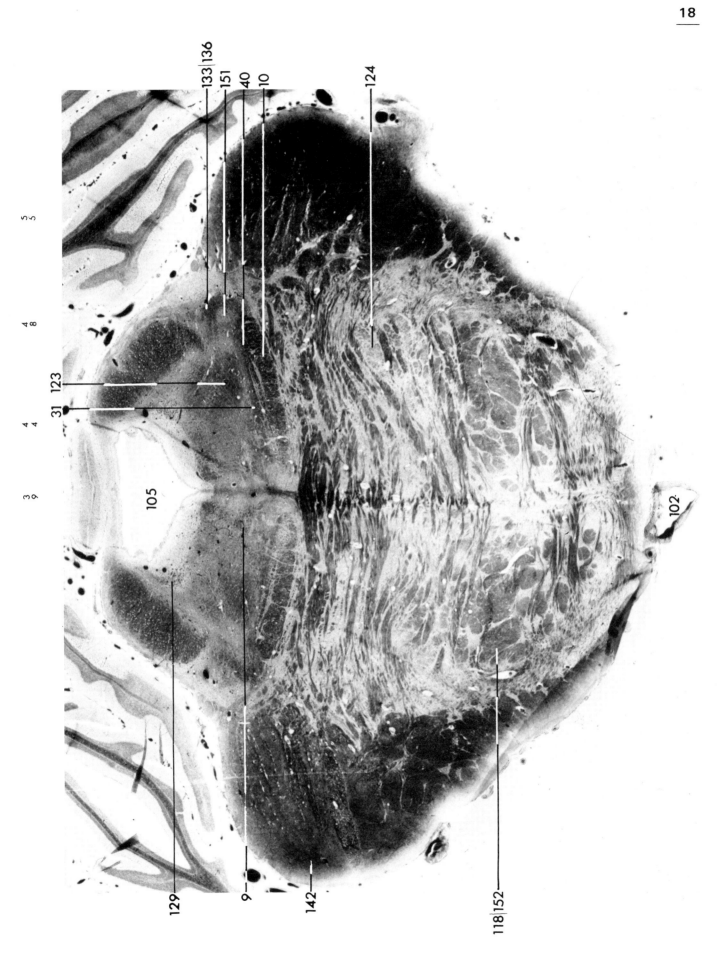

FIGURE 19.

Rostral Pons at the Junction with the Mesencephalon

The sagittal photograph before Figure 1 shows the extent to which Figure 19 and later figures deviate from the transverse plane. Although, dorsally, Figure 19 includes the extreme rostral end of the pons and a small portion of the overhanging edge of the inferior colliculus (209), ventrally, almost half of the basilar pons still lies rostral to this figure. A number of factors contribute to this: the basilar and tegmental pons together form a structure that is much broader ventrally than dorsally (Fig. 39); moreover, the persistence of the cephalic flexure, which appears during embryologic development, leaves the mesencephalon and the prosencephalon set at an angle with reference to the caudal brain stem. If true transverse sections of the rostral brain stem had been made, a large wedge of ventral pons would necessarily have been eliminated from the consecutive series of slides.

The decussation of the trochlear nerve (203) occurs dorsally in the rostral end of the anterior medullary velum. Since the nucleus (208, Fig. 42) lies ventral to the cerebral aqueduct at the transverse level of the inferior colliculus, the root fibers not only must follow a semicircular course around the cerebral aqueduct but also must extend caudally in order to emerge from the brain at the caudal edge of the inferior colliculus. Although the trochlear nucleus (208) appears to lie ventral to the superior colliculus (210) in Figure 21, this appearance is due to the oblique plane of section.

The superior cerebellar peduncle (211) is no longer in the lateral edge of the anterior medullary velum as it was in previous sections. Instead, it has now entered the tegmentum of the pons in a course which is directed rostrally, ventrally, and medially toward the decussation of the superior cerebellar pe-

duncles (200, Figs. 21 to 23). This decussation is at the transverse level of the inferior colliculus (Fig. 40). Readjustments in the positions of the great ascending systems of suprasegmental fibers are related to this shift in the superior cerebellar peduncle. The fibers of the lateral lemniscus (136) are directed rostrally. In order to reach their major synapse in the inferior colliculus, they pass dorsally and to the lateral side of the superior cerebellar peduncle as the latter plunges into the tegmentum of the pons. Spinothalamic fibers, which are dispersed in the lateral lemniscus, follow the same general course but do not, of course, synapse in the inferior colliculus. The shift of the medial lemniscus (10) laterally in the pons has just begun. A little further rostral, it too follows the lateral lemniscus in an oblique course across the lateral side of the superior cerebellar peduncle in its approach to the thalamus (10, Figs. 21 to 27). The relative positions of the medial longitudinal fasciculus (8) and central tegmental tract (123) are unchanged.

The plane of section is now rostral to all but a trace of the middle cerebellar peduncle.

8—Medial longitudinal fasciculus
10—Medial lemniscus
31—Ventral central trigeminal tract
40—Rubrospinal tract
103—Pontocerebellar fibers
104—Pontine nuclei
123—Central tegmental tract
124—Corticopontine fibers
129—Mesencephalic nucleus and tract of the trigeminal nerve
133—Lateral spinothalamic tract
136—Lateral lemniscus
150—Trigeminal nerve
203—Decussation of the trochlear nerve
209—Inferior colliculus
211—Superior cerebellar peduncle

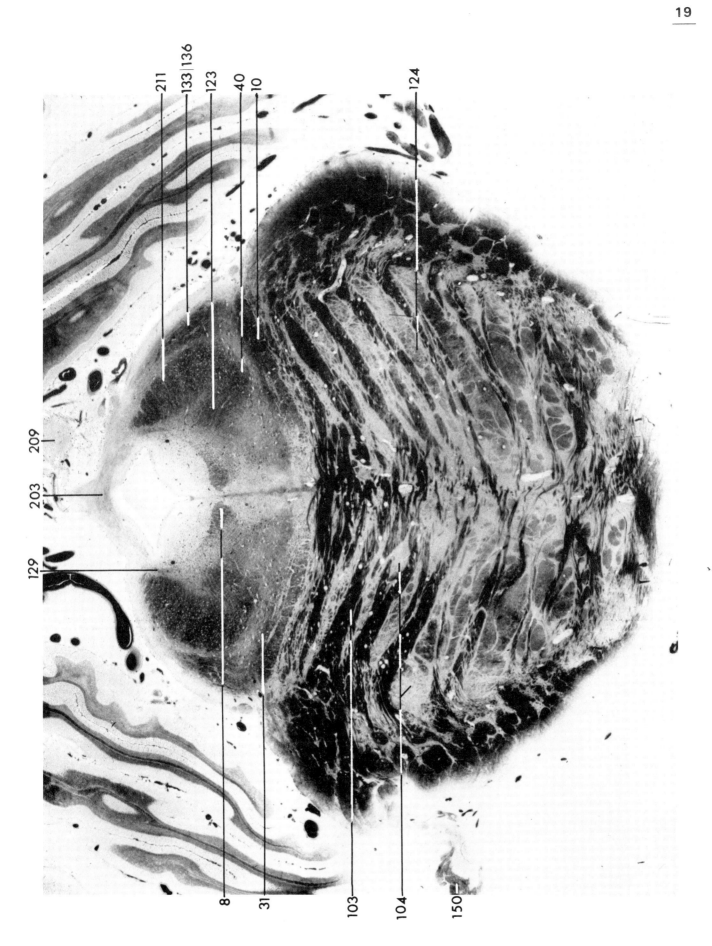

FIGURE 20. Upper Pons and Inferior Colliculi

In the rostral pons, corticospinal fibers (118) are widely dispersed and no longer resemble the pyramids, as they did in the caudal pons. In addition, they are also intermingled with corticobulbar fibers to the somatic and branchiomeric motor nuclei, which innervate striated muscles controlled by cranial nerves. Indeed, all the descending suprasegmental fibers in the basilar pons are more or less interdigitated, although it is reasonably safe to label the lateral transected fibers as corticopontine fibers (124), since they can be followed rostrally into the lateral side of the crus cerebri (220, Fig. 21), where corticopontine fibers are rather sharply segregated.

Not all corticobulbar fibers are contained in the basilar portion of the pons: beginning in the rostral mesencephalon (Fig. 28), corticobulbar fibers continually disperse into the tegmentum of the mesencephalon, pons, and medulla, where they take a variety of atypical and aberrant routes, both crossed and direct. Some descend in the medial longitudinal fasciculus (8) and medial lemniscus (10). Pick's bundle (39, Figs. 8 to 11) is an example of aberrant corticobulbar fibers. These accompany corticospinal fibers to the decussation of the pyramids, where they become sharply recurrent and ascend as Pick's bundle to synapse in motor nuclei. Because of the various courses corticobulbar fibers may take, it can be difficult to localize the site of a lesion of them within the brain stem. In addition, some cranial nerve motor nuclei are innervated by corticobulbar fibers arising in both hemispheres, and there may be no obvious paralysis after a unilateral lesion of these fibers.

In the tegmentum of the mesencephalon, the lateral lemniscus (136) is sectioned midway in its oblique course across the lateral side of the superior cerebellar peduncle (211) to its major termination in the inferior colliculus (209). The lateral spinothalamic tract (133) is dispersed in the lateral lemniscus.

The medial lemniscus (10) and probably the ventral central trigeminal tract (31) have shifted only slightly laterally in comparison with the previous figure.

The reticular formation is reduced in area in the mesencephalon and is largely obscured by the central tegmental tract (123) and the superior cerebellar peduncle (211), which are intermingled. The figure includes just a little of the caudal edge of the decussation of the superior cerebellar peduncles (200).

The tectum, being that part of the mesencephalon dorsal to the cerebral aqueduct, here includes the two inferior colliculi (209). Most of the auditory fibers of the lateral lemniscus (136) synapse in this nucleus. The few which do not are found to extend directly into the brachium of the inferior colliculus (222, Fig. 21). The inferior colliculus is both a relay nucleus in the auditory pathway and a center for reflexes initiated by sound. Some fibers emerge from it and descend to relay nuclei of the auditory system, but most axons ascend as the brachium of the inferior colliculus (222, Fig. 21). The brachium can be followed to its termination in the medial geniculate nucleus (333, Fig. 23), which is still another of the relay nuclei in the auditory pathway to the cerebral cortex.

Ventral to the inferior colliculi are the root fibers of the trochlear nerve (212). This is the only nerve which decussates completely and which emerges on the dorsal surface of the brain stem.

40—Rubrospinal tract
102—Basilar artery
118—Corticospinal fibers
123—Central tegmental tract
124—Corticopontine fibers
133—Lateral spinothalamic tract
136—Lateral lemniscus
150—Trigeminal nerve
152—Corticobulbar fibers
200—Decussation of the superior
      cerebellar peduncles
209—Inferior colliculus
211—Superior cerebellar peduncle
212—Trochlear fibers

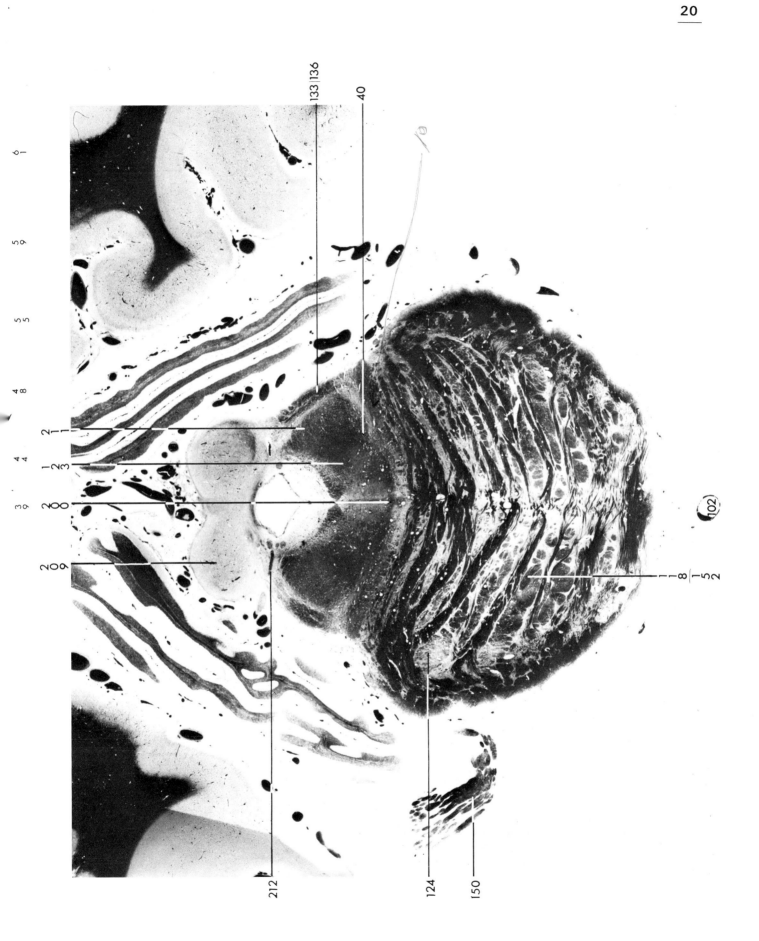

FIGURE 21.

Levels of the Superior and Inferior Colliculi and Pons

This oblique section includes the rostral basilar pons and both rostral and caudal parts of the mesencephalon. The tectum containing the superior colliculi (210) is rostral mesencephalon. The tegmentum is caudal mesencephalon since it includes the decussation of the superior cerebellar peduncles (200) and the trochlear nucleus (208). The crus cerebri (220) which occupies the most ventral part of the mesencephalon is only just included in the section, far laterally. Corticopontine fibers constitute the lateral part of the crus. Their continuity with those in the basilar pons is obvious.

Changes in the position of the great ascending systems of sensory fibers are of major interest. Most auditory fibers constituting the lateral lemniscus have terminated in the inferior colliculus (209, Fig. 20), although a few axons bypassed this synapse and have entered the brachium of the inferior colliculus (222). However, most of the ascending axons in this brachium arise in the inferior colliculus. Both groups of fibers terminate in the medial geniculate nucleus (333, Fig. 23).

Medial to the brachium of the inferior colliculus is a larger, semicircular accumulation of fibers in the lateral and ventral part of the tegmentum of the mesencephalon. The fibers most ventral and medial are, indubitably, those of position and tactile sensibility in the medial lemniscus (10), while those medial to the brachium of the inferior colliculus are, indubitably, fibers of the lateral spinothalamic tract (133) and the ventral central trigeminal tract (31). However, there is some mingling of these tracts in the intermediate portion of the semicircular band of fibers. Apparently, in its ascent the ventral central trigeminal tract shifts laterally and dorsally, thereby departing from its relationship with the medial lemniscus in the pons

to mingle with fibers of the lateral spinothalamic tract at the level of the mesencephalon.

Two portions of the thalamus are present. The pineal gland (308) is representative of the epithalamus, while the pulvinar (324) is part of the dorsal thalamus. On either side of the pineal gland are the internal cerebral veins (452), which convey blood from the deep central regions of the thalamus and cerebrum to the great cerebral vein of Galen, and by it to the straight sinus. The large, engorged arteries in the subarachnoid space around the brain stem are the superior cerebellar and the posterior cerebral arteries, penultimate and terminal branches, respectively, of the basilar artery (102, Fig. 20).

The *leader* to the central tegmental tract (123) crosses a lightly stained area of reticular formation occupied by the pedunculopontine nucleus. In Figure 22 only that portion of the *leader* is black. This nucleus is the most caudal terminus for descending extrapyramidal fibers that originate in the globus pallidus. Additional pertinent comment accompanies Figure 30.

8—Medial longitudinal fasciculus
10—Medial lemniscus
31—Ventral central trigeminal tract
40—Rubrospinal tract
104—Pontine nuclei
123—Central tegmental tract
133—Lateral spinothalamic tract
200—Decussation of the superior cerebellar peduncles
205—Cerebral aqueduct
208—Trochlear nucleus
210—Superior colliculus
215—Periaqueductal gray matter
220—Crus cerebri (pes pedunculi)
222—Brachium of the inferior colliculus
308—Pineal body
324—Pulvinar
400—Splenium of the corpus callosum
430—Major forceps of the corpus callosum
452—Internal cerebral veins

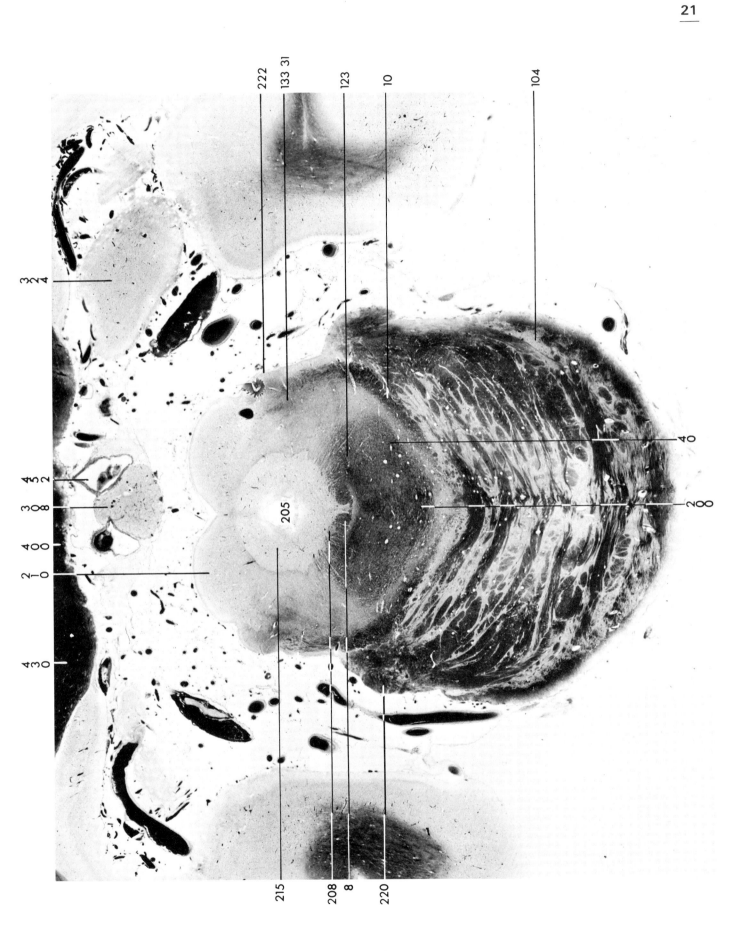

222

133 31

123

10

104

32

45 2

38

40

210

43

205

40

20

215

208 8

220

FIGURE 22.

Level of the Superior Colliculus and the Caudal Diencephalon

It is obvious that the dorsal brain stem in this figure still resembles that of Figure 21. In the ventral and lateral part of the tegmentum of the mesencephalon, the medial lemniscus (10), the lateral spinothalamic (133) and ventral central trigeminal (31) tracts, and the brachium of the inferior colliculus (222) form a continuous area of fibers. This is the only level of the brain stem at which the position of the ventral central trigeminal tract is documented by much evidence. Surgeons who made a shallow transverse incision to sever the lateral spinothalamic tract (133) at this level reported contralateral analgesia, not only of the body but also of the face. It is postulated that the ventral central trigeminal tract, which may be in close relation to the dorsal part of the medial lemniscus in the pons (Fig. 17), shifts laterally in ascent and so comes close to or mingles with the lateral spinothalamic tract in the mesencephalon. Apparently the localization of fibers is such that the body is represented upside down because it was found that, unless the incision extended well up the slope of the superior colliculus, the contralateral inferior part of the body remained sensitive when the upper part was analgesic. Although the brachium of the inferior colliculus is also severed in this operation (mesencephalic tractotomy), hearing is only slightly affected, if at all, because auditory impulses are conducted bilaterally.

The tegmentum ventral to the cerebral aqueduct (205) shows the structures present at the level of the inferior colliculus in a true transverse section. Major among these are the trochlear nucleus (208) and the massive decussation of the superior cerebellar peduncles (200). Most of the peduncular fibers ascend to the red nucleus (214, Fig. 25), intermediate ventral (337, Fig. 31) and anterior ventral (329, Fig. 36) thalamic nuclei and small intralaminar nuclei within the internal medullary lamina of the thalamus (339, Figs. 30 to 34). Some peduncular fibers descend and synapse in reticular nuclei in the brain stem.

The rubrospinal fibers (40), which occupy a lateral position in the spinal cord (Figs. 4 to 6) and lower brain stem (Fig. 16), are gradually moving medially toward their origin in the red nucleus.

More of the crus cerebri (220) is included here than in the previous section. Several different fiber tracts are contained within the crus cerebri, but only the corticospinal (118) and corticobulbar (152) fibers are labeled. The lateral edge of the crus contains corticopontine fibers.

The dentate gyrus (439) and hippocampus (432) are two of the oldest derivatives of the telencephalon. These two areas of cortical gray matter extend rostrally from this level and will become more prominent in Figures 23 to 29, along with the fornix. Axons originating in the hippocampus collect to form the fimbria of the hippocampus (440), which at first courses caudally. Just about at the present level the fimbria makes a hair pin dorsal turn and now, as the crus of the fornix (410), extends rostrally. In the following figures the fornix gradually approaches the midline and extends forward, ventral to the corpus callosum (Figs. 23 to 38). At the level represented in Figure 38, the fibers recurve and course caudally to terminate in part in the mamillary nuclei (300, Fig. 31). The fornix is a major efferent tract from the limbic system. Its specific function is not well established. Afferent fibers to the dentate gyrus and hippocampus arise in part in the parahippocampal gyrus (431), formerly known as the hippocampal gyrus and therefore frequently confused with the hippocampus itself.

There are many blood vessels in the space between the brain stem and the pulvinar of the thalamus (324). The larger ones, not labeled, are the posterior cerebral and superior cerebellar arteries, the terminal and paraterminal branches, respectively, of the basilar artery (102, Fig. 39). These two arteries follow close, parallel courses around the brain stem (125 and 407, Figs. 44 to 57) and vascularize the dorsal and lateral parts of the brain stem shown here, in addition to the regions of the cerebrum and cerebellum suggested by their names. These vessels complicate the mesencephalic tractotomy for the relief of pain referred to above.

31—Ventral central trigeminal tract
40—Rubrospinal tract
118—Corticospinal tract
123—Central tegmental tract
133—Lateral spinothalamic tract
152—Corticobulbar fibers
200—Decussation of the superior cerebellar peduncles
208—Trochlear nucleus
215—Periaqueductal gray matter
222—Brachium of the inferior colliculus
406—Body of the lateral ventricle
408—Tela choroidea of the lateral ventricle
410—Crus of the fornix
430—Major forceps of the corpus callosum
431—Parahippocampal gyrus (hippocampal gyrus)
432—Hippocampus
439—Dentate gyrus
440—Fimbria of the hippocampus

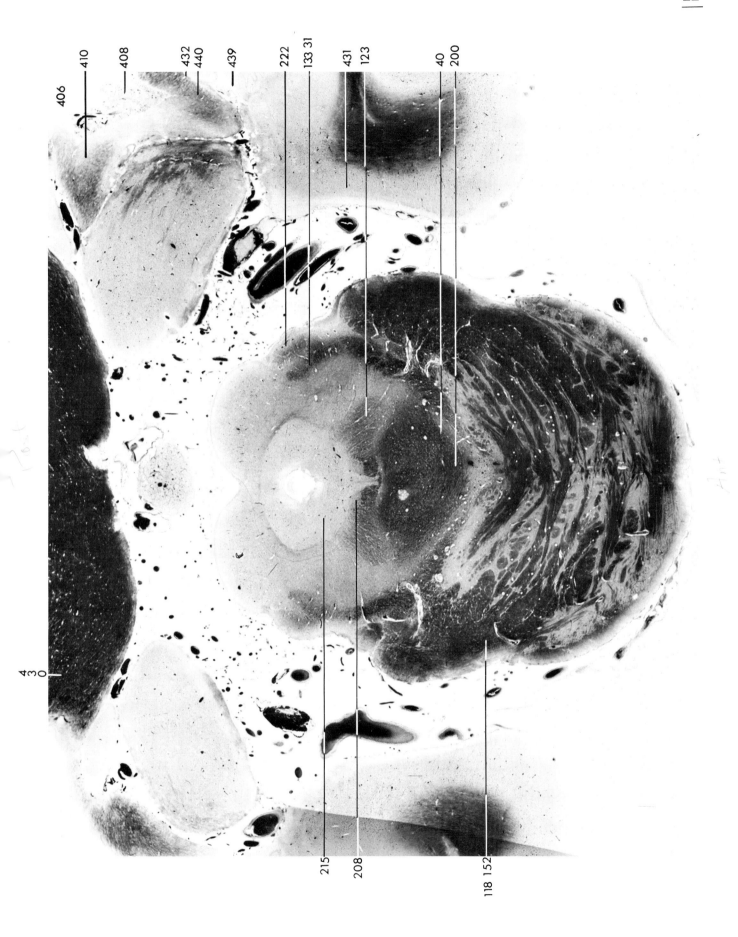

406 410 408 432 440 439 222 133 31 431 123 40 200

4 3 0

215 208 118 152

FIGURE 23. Junction of the Mesencephalon and Thalamus TRANSVERSE

The continuity between mesencephalon and diencephalon is established dorsally, while ventrally the rostral end of the pons is still included. Most of the fibers in the superior cerebellar peduncles (211) have crossed at more caudal levels of the decussation (200) and are now directed toward terminations in the red nucleus (214, Fig. 25) and several thalamic nuclei. Dorsal to the peduncle, the medial longitudinal fasciculus (8) is not distinct from the central tegmental tract (123) along its lateral edge. The oculomotor complex of nuclei (201) occupies the ventral part of the periaqueductal gray matter (215). These nuclei contain the cell bodies of axons to many of the extraocular muscles and the cell bodies of the parasympathetic preganglionic fibers that control the sphincter of the iris and the ciliary muscle. Oculomotor fibers (207) are visible in the substantia nigra (221), close to where they emerge in the interpeduncular fossa (206, Fig. 24). Laterally, in the tegmentum of the mesencephalon, the great ascending sensory tracts from the body and face form a continuous band of fibers which is labeled regionally as the medial lemniscus (10), the lateral spinothalamic tract (133), and the ventral central trigeminal tract (31). The auditory fibers, which form the brachium of the inferior colliculus (222), are entering the medial side of the medial geniculate nucleus (333); from this nucleus issue axons collectively called auditory radiations (442, Fig. 25), which extend to the transverse temporal gyri of the cerebral cortex, where sound is perceived.

The fibers arching dorsally over the medial geniculate nucleus constitute the brachium of the superior colliculus (223). Cell bodies of axons in the brachium are located in the ganglion layer of the retina, and their fibers course successively through the optic nerve, chiasm, and tract (314, 302, and 328, Fig. 34) to terminate in the superior colliculus (210) and pretectal area (218, Fig. 24). The optic tract can be followed in the sections from Figure 34 caudally. In Figure 25 some of the axons of the optic tract pass to the medial side of the lateral geniculate body to become the brachium of the superior colliculus (223). The superior colliculus is the center for light reflexes mediated by skeletal muscle (turning of the head and eyes), while the pretectal area mediates reflexes involving smooth muscle (pupillary light reflex).

The lateral geniculate nucleus (338) is a thalamic nucleus which relays sensory impulses to the cerebral cortex. It too receives impulses initiated by light which are propagated along fibers in the optic nerve, chiasm, and tract. From the lateral geniculate nucleus axons extend in the geniculocalcarine tract to the occipital cerebral cortex, where light and color are perceived. The tract is located here in the ventral part of the retrolenticular part of the internal capsule (444), immediately dorsal and lateral to the lateral geniculate nucleus. In the functional classification of thalamic nuclei, both the medial and the lateral geniculate nuclei are cortical relay nuclei, since they convey impulses initiated in peripheral receptors to the cerebral cortex.

Dorsal to the geniculate nuclei is the pulvinar (324). The pulvinar does not receive direct sensory information via suprasegmental fiber tracts, as do the geniculate nuclei. Instead, its major afferent connections are with other thalamic nuclei and with the cerebral cortex. Impulses are said to be associated within this large nucleus and then propagated to the cerebral cortex via fibers in the internal capsule. Hence the pulvinar is classified as an associational thalamic nucleus. Its functions are not specifically known. However, its cortical connections are with areas that are thought to be concerned with an integration of impulses initiated by light and color, and with the recognition of objects and language symbols.

The internal capsule is a large accumulation of fibers, both afferent and efferent with respect to the cerebrum. It is present in all remaining sections in this transverse series. The portion in this figure is the retrolenticular part of the internal capsule (444), so named because it is caudal to the lentiform nucleus, the general name for the globus pallidus and putamen (421 and 419, Fig. 30). The internal capsule occupies the region where, during development, the cerebral hemisphere grows caudally along the lateral side of the thalamus and fuses with it. The area of fusion is secondarily invaded by axons of thalamic neurons extending to the cerebral cortex and by axons issuing from the cerebral cortex to form corticospinal, corticopontine, and corticothalamic tracts, among others. Corticospinal and corticopontine fibers continue as constituents of the crus cerebri (220); in the following figures the physical continuity between the crus cerebri and the internal capsule can be verified (Figs. 24 to 26). However, the retrolenticular portion of the internal capsule contains no corticospinal and only a few corticopontine fibers. Instead, the retrolenticular internal capsule consists in large part of reciprocal connections between caudal thalamic nuclei and caudal cerebral cortex. Among these, major ones are the auditory and optic radiations.

8—Medial longitudinal fasciculus
10—Medial lemniscus
31—Ventral central trigeminal tract
123—Central tegmental tract
133—Lateral spinothalamic tract
200—Decussation of the superior cerebellar peduncles
201—Oculomotor nucleus
205—Cerebral aqueduct
207—Oculomotor fibers
210—Superior colliculus
211—Superior cerebellar peduncle
220—Crus cerebri (pes pedunculi)
221—Substantia nigra
222—Brachium of the inferior colliculus
223—Brachium of the superior colliculus
225—Interstitial nucleus
226—Nucleus of Darkschewitsch
308—Pineal body
324—Pulvinar
333—Medial geniculate nucleus
338—Lateral geniculate nucleus
400—Splenium of the corpus callosum
408—Tela choroidea of the lateral ventricle
426—Inferior horn of the lateral ventricle
440—Fimbria of the hippocampus
444—Retrolenticular part of the internal capsule
452—Internal cerebral veins
453—Strionigral and pallidotegmental fibers
455—Vena and stria terminalis

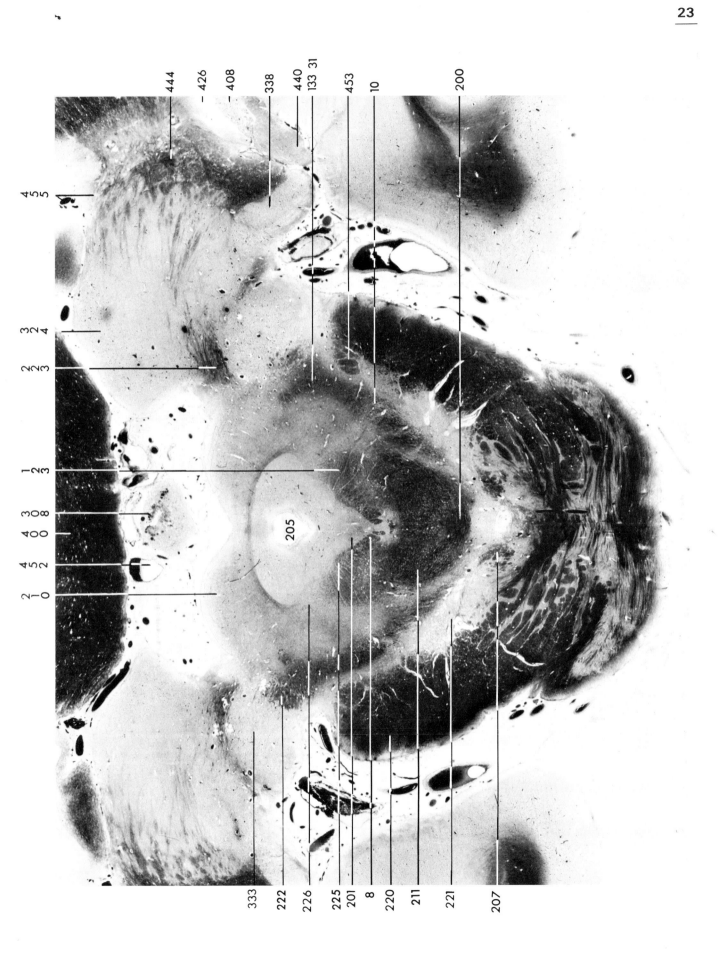

FIGURE 24. Junction of the Mesencephalon and Pons

Dorsal to the cerebral aqueduct, the plane of section passes through an ill defined region in the rostral slope of the superior colliculus called the pretectal area (218). A few fibers of the brachium of the superior colliculus (223) are labeled where they enter it. The pretectal area is a center for light reflexes mediated by the autonomic nervous system. From this center and from the center in the superior colliculus, axons arise which cross ventral to the oculomotor nucleus (201) in the dorsal tegmental decussation (229), descend as the tectospinal tract (9, Figs. 18 to 9) in the brain stem to enter the spinal cord as a constituent of the medial longitudinal fasciculus. The optic tract (328), which approaches the lateral geniculate nucleus (338) from the rostral direction, is just beginning to be included in the section. As previously noted, it is the fibers which by-pass a synapse in the lateral geniculate nucleus that constitute the brachium of the superior colliculus. Immediately lateral to the lateral geniculate nucleus is the retrolenticular part of the internal capsule (444), a major constituent of which is the geniculocalcarine tract. This tract conveys impulses initiated in the eye from the lateral geniculate nucleus to the medial surface of the occipital cerebral cortex, where they are perceived as light and color. Some of the fibers covering the dorsolateral side of the medial geniculate nucleus are fibers constituting the auditory radiations, with cell bodies in the medial geniculate nucleus. These axons also extend laterally, enter the internal capsule, and ultimately terminate in the anterior transverse temporal gyri, where the impulses they propagate are perceived as sound.

The great ascending sensory tracts, the medial lemniscus (10), the spinothalamic tract (133), and the ventral central trigeminal tract (31), are now indistinguishably blended as they approach their termination in the posterior ventral thalamic nuclei (332 and 336, Fig. 27).

The ventral tegmental decussation (224) marks the crossing of axons arising in the red nucleus (214, Fig. 25). Further caudal these fibers are identified as the rubrospinal tract. Rubroreticular fibers also cross in the ventral tegmental decussation and descend to synapse in nuclei of the reticular formation. The impulses both tracts convey ultimately converge upon motor nuclei of the cranial and spinal nerves.

Only the extreme rostral tip of the basilar pons is still included in the section. There are many branches of the posterior medial striate arteries (202) in the interpeduncular fossa (206), and the oculomotor nerve (217) is just entering it. The full width of the crus cerebri (220) is now visible. The medial and lateral ends of each crus contain corticopontine fibers, which enter the basilar pons and synapse in pontine nuclei, as already seen. The central portion of a crus is occupied by corticobulbar fibers medially and corticospinal fibers laterally. Furthermore, corticospinal fibers affecting the upper extremity are localized medial to those affecting the lower extremity. A crossed paralysis (Weber's syndrome) results when a vascular lesion which involves branches of the posterior medial striate arteries interrupts conduction in the ipsilateral axons of the oculomotor nucleus (lower motor neurons) and the corticospinal fibers (upper motor neurons) in the crus cerebri. Since the corticospinal fibers cross in the decussation of the pyramids (4, Figs. 7 and 40), the motor impairment is in the contralateral side of the body which, with the ipsilateral ocular impairment, results in a crossed or alternating paralysis.

Comment on the cerebral ventricular system and adnexa is appropriate. The body (406) and the tela choroidea (408) of the lateral ventricle are labeled in the dorsal part of the section. Just dorsal to the alveus (433) is the inferior horn of the lateral ventricle and

its tela choroidea (426 and 408, Fig. 26). Axons of neurons which are for the most part in the hippocampus (432) converge first to form the tract of fibers in the floor of the inferior horn of the lateral ventricle called the alveus (433), which continue as the fimbria of the fornix (440). The recurrent course of the fimbria to form the crus of the fornix (410) is illustrated in Figure 22. The fornix can be followed to a major termination in the mamillary body (300, Fig. 31). The rostral end of the fornix also follows a recurrent course before ending in a mamillary body. One or another of the subdivisions of the fornix occurs in every one of the remaining figures in the transverse series. In some sections here and rostrally, the fornix is transected twice, where it is recurrent near its origin and termination. Note how the fornix forms the medial wall of both the inferior horn and the body of the lateral ventricle.

10—Medial lemniscus
31—Ventral central trigeminal tract
123—Central tegmental tract
133—Lateral spinothalamic tract
201—Oculomotor nucleus
202—Posteromedial striate arteries
206—Interpeduncular fossa
211—Superior cerebellar peduncle
217—**Oculomotor nerve**
218—Pretectal area
223—Brachium of the superior colliculus
224—Ventral tegmental decussation
229—Dorsal tegmental decussation
328—Optic tract
338—Medial geniculate nucleus
338—Lateral geniculate nucleus
406—Body of the lateral ventricle
408—Tela choroidea of the lateral ventricle
410—Crus of the fornix
431—Parahippocampal gyrus (hippocampal gyrus)
432—Hippocampus
433—Alveus
444—Retrolenticular part of the internal capsule
453—Strionigral and pallidotegmental fibers

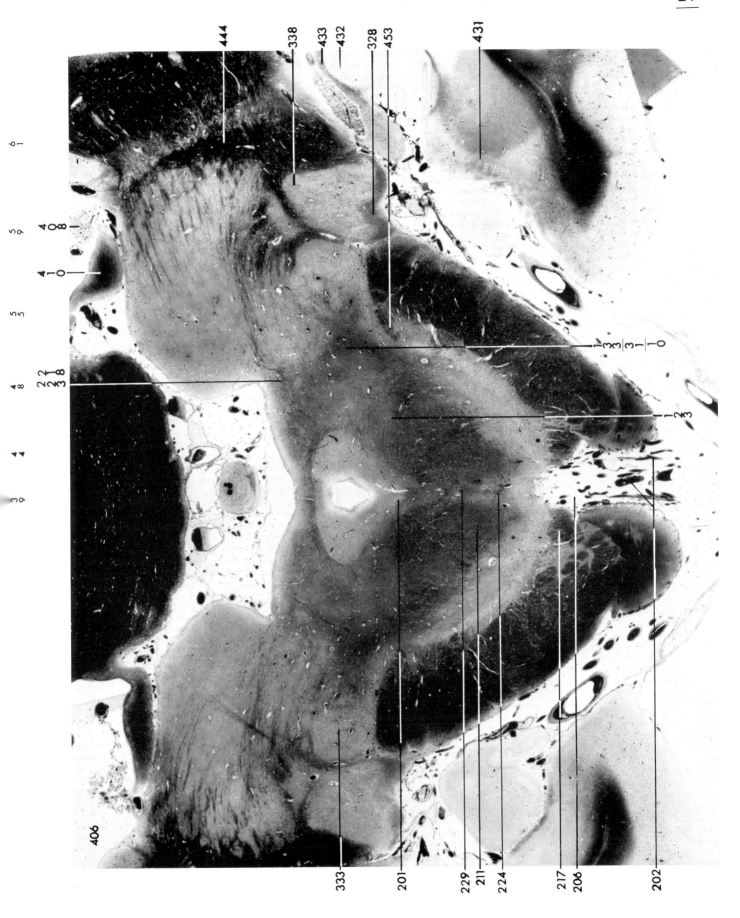

FIGURE 25. Junction of Mesencephalon and Pons

Except for the inclusion here of the red nucleus, this figure resembles the previous one. This nucleus receives impulses from the dentate, emboliform, and globose nuclei (137, 130, and 126, Fig. 14) via axons coursing in the superior cerebellar peduncle. Other axons arising in these nuclei pass beyond the red nucleus as the cerebellothalamic tract (219) and synapse in the intermediate ventral, anterior ventral, and intralaminar nuclei. The intermediate and anterior ventral nuclei have reciprocal connections, via the internal capsule, with that part of the frontal lobe most directly related to volitional movements.

Since the medial longitudinal fasciculus (8) does not extend rostrally beyond the level of the posterior commissure (309) and pretectal area (218), as is evident in Figure 39 of the sagittal series, Figure 25 is the last cross section to show the medial longitudinal fasciculus. This fasciculus disappears, because most of the ascending fibers in the medial longitudinal fasciculus terminate in the motor nuclei of the trochlear and oculomotor nuclei, and in the nucleus of Darkschewitsch (226, Fig. 23), while most descending fibers do not arise from nuclei more rostral than the interstitial nucleus (225, Fig. 23).

The central tegmental (123) is another vanishing tract because most of its descending fibers originate here and at lower levels of the brain stem, while ascending fibers are spreading out to several terminations. The ascending fibers are important. These originate in reticular nuclei of the pons and medulla, and upon entering the diencephalon at about this level they diverge from the tract into the subthalamus and into the intralaminar and reticular nuclei of the thalamus. They cannot be followed in these figures. Another group of fibers which arise in reticular nuclei in the mesencephalon send axons into the hypothalamus (343, Fig. 30) via the mamillary peduncle. The peduncle (not labeled) is probably located just ventral and lateral to the ventral tegmental decussation (224). All of these fibers appear to be part of the ascending reticular activating system, which has important effects upon the neural activity of the cerebral cortex and upon behavior.

The proximity of the medial and lateral geniculate nuclei (333 and 338) and the retrolenticular part of the internal capsule (444) illustrate the ease with which the auditory (442) and optic radiations can become incorporated in it.

While the posterior commissure is a large tract, its connections are not fully known. Axons from the pretectal area (218), such as those which mediate the consensual pupillary light reflex, extend through it to the contralateral oculomotor nucleus, specifically, to that portion giving origin to parasympathetic, preganglionic fibers. Reciprocal fibers between the superior colliculi also cross in the posterior commissure.

8—Medial longitudinal fasciculus
10—Medial lemniscus
31—Ventral central trigeminal tract
123—Central tegmental tract
133—Lateral spinothalamic tract
205—Cerebral aqueduct
206—Interpeduncular fossa
207—Oculomotor fibers
214—Red nucleus
218—Pretectal area
219—Cerebellothalamic (dentatothalamic) tract
220—Crus cerebri (pes pedunculi)
221—Substantia nigra
222—Brachium of the inferior colliculus
223—Brachium of the superior colliculus
224—Ventral tegmental decussation
229—Dorsal tegmental decussation
309—Posterior commissure
324—Pulvinar
333—Medial geniculate nucleus
338—Lateral geniculate nucleus
400—Splenium of the corpus callosum
432—Hippocampus
433—Alveus
439—Dentate gyrus
440—Fimbria of the hippocampus
442—Auditory radiations
443—Tail of the caudate nucleus
444—Retrolenticular part of the internal capsule
452—Internal cerebral veins
453—Strionigral and pallidotegmental fibers
455—Stria and vena terminalis

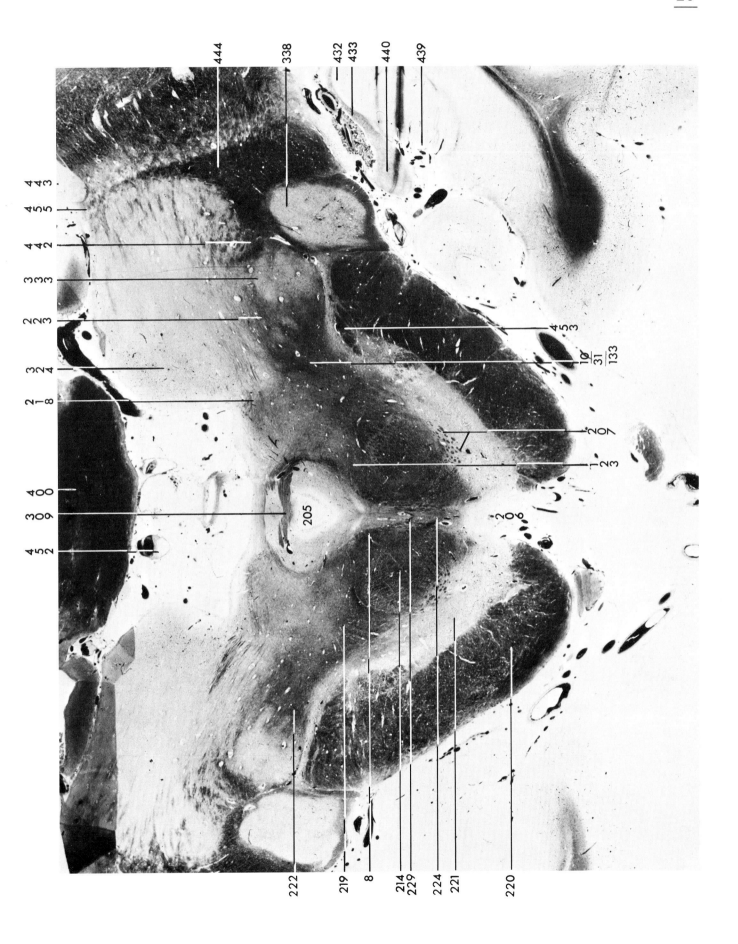

FIGURE 26. Red Nucleus and Caudal Thalamus

The plane of this section is immediately rostral to the lateral geniculate nuclei, and the figure includes oblique sections of the optic tracts (328) which, in Figures 24 and 25, were seen only as myelinated fibers along the ventral aspect of a lateral geniculate nucleus. The optic tract is present in the sections from here rostrally to its origin in the optic chiasm (302, Fig. 34). Throughout its course it is a landmark which arbitrarily separates the internal capsule (444) and the crus cerebri (220). The axons in the two are, of course, continuous; only the name changes.

The ventricular system of the brain stem is now enlarging as the cerebral aqueduct of Figure 25 expands into the third ventricle (307) here. Dorsal to it and to the posterior commissure (309) are the habenular nuclei (315). Each habenular nucleus gives origin to axons which constitute the fasciculus retroflexus (318) and which terminate in the interpeduncular nucleus (213, Fig. 27). The large size of the fasciculus is apparent in the following figure. Some impulses from the habenula are propagated caudally and reach general visceral efferent cranial nerve nuclei via the dorsal longitudinal fasciculus (5, Fig. 11) or the reticular formation or both. Habenular nuclei receive axons, via the stria medullaris of the thalamus (316, Figs. 34 to 28), which convey impulses initiated in the olfactory nerve by odors. These impulses traverse an intricate series of nuclei and fiber tracts before entering the stria medullaris. Hence, by this devious chain—stria medullaris of the thalamus, habenular nucleus, fasciculus retroflexus, interpeduncular nucleus, dorsal longitudinal fasciculus, and several visceral efferent nuclei—visceral responses to olfactory stimuli can occur. It is not indubitably established that axons of the interpeduncular nucleus enter the dorsal longitudinal fasciculus or the reticular formation. Moreover, the functions of this intricate series of neurons remain vague, despite the impressive size of the fasciculus retroflexus.

The thalamic reticular nucleus (340) is becoming prominent along the dorsolateral edge of the thalamus. It is separated from the rest of the thalamus by the external medullary lamina (334). This nucleus lies along the entire lateral aspect of the thalamus, as far rostral as the anterior ventral nucleus (329, Fig. 36). The reticular nucleus has connections with many other thalamic nuclei and with reticular nuclei of the brain stem, but no fibers project to the cerebral cortex. The vague function of integration has been suggested for it.

10—Medial lemniscus
31—Ventral central trigeminal tract
133—Lateral spinothalamic tract
206—Interpeduncular fossa
207—Oculomotor fibers
219—Cerebellothalamic (dentatothalamic) tract
307—Third ventricle
309—Posterior commissure
315—Habenula
318—Fasciculus retroflexus
328—Optic tract
334—External medullary lamina of the thalamus
340—Reticular nuclei of the thalamus
406—Body of the lateral ventricle
408—Tela choroidea of the lateral ventricle
410—Crus of the fornix
426—Inferior horn of the lateral ventricle
431—Parahippocampal gyrus (hippocampal gyrus)
432—Hippocampus
433—Alveus
439—Dentate gyrus
440—Fimbria of the hippocampus
444—Retrolenticular part of the internal capsule
454—Uncinate gyrus

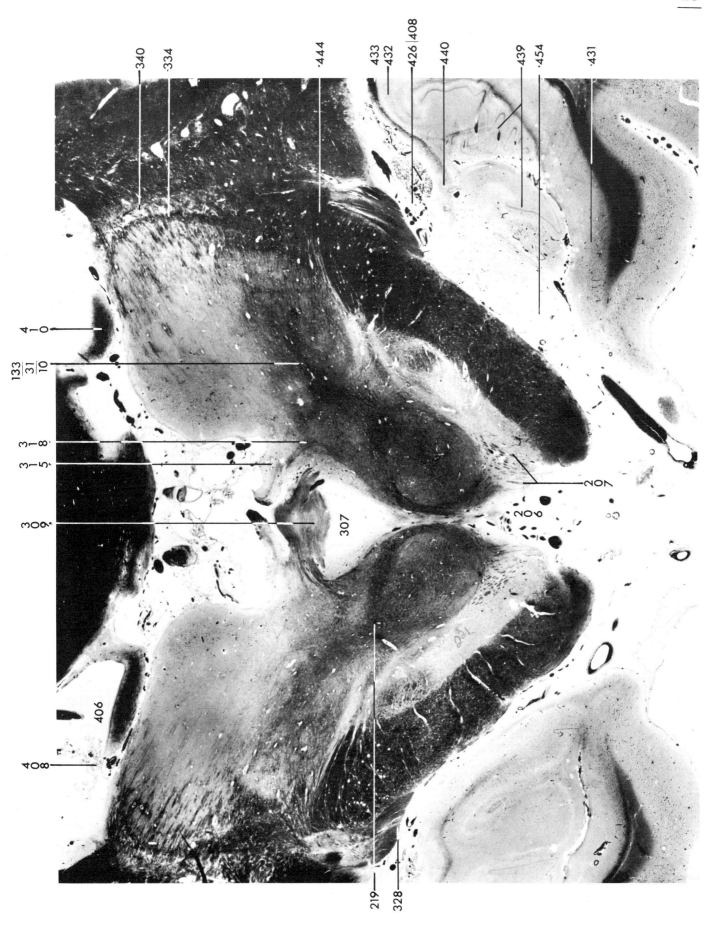

340
334
444
433
432
426 408
440
439
454
431

4
1
0

133
31
10

3 3
1 8

3 3
5 5

3
0 9

307

207

206

406

4
0 8

219
328

FIGURE 27.

Junction of the Mesencephalon and Diencephalon

Two specific thalamic relay nuclei, the posteromedial ventral (332) and the posterolateral ventral (336) nuclei are cardinal new features of this section. Ventral to them, in the mélange of myelinated fibers, are the ascending sensory fibers of the lemniscal systems (10, 31, and 133), the cerebellothalamic tract (219), and the rubrothalamic tract (230). Those lemniscal fibers which originate chiefly in the superior sensory and spinal nuclei of the trigeminal nerve and which traverse trigeminal tracts (31) synapse in the posteromedial ventral nucleus. Fibers in the medial lemniscus (10) and the lateral spinothalamic tract (133), which convey similar general sensory impulses but from the body rather than the face, synapse in the posterolateral ventral nucleus. Both nuclei in turn project fibers to the postcentral gyrus of the cerebrum. These can be seen immediately lateral to the two principal specific thalamic relay nuclei (332 and 336) where many axons traverse the reticular nucleus (340), thereby obscuring it, to enter the posterior limb of the internal capsule (418). Mingled with these corticipetal fibers are corticothalamic fibers from the somesthetic area in the postcentral gyrus to the posteromedial ventral and posterolateral ventral thalamic nuclei (332 and 336).

The cerebellothalamic (219) and perhaps a rubrothalamic tract (230) extend rostrally beyond this figure to synapse chiefly in the intermediate ventral, anterior ventral, and some intralaminar nuclei. The anterior ventral and intermediate ventral are cortical relay nuclei since their axons project impulses of cerebellar origin to the cerebral cortex.

There are also descending fibers in the myelinated area where the ascending lemniscal systems are labeled. Most of these arise in the globus pallidus. They project to reticular nuclei in the mesencephalon and possibly to the substantia nigra. Strionigral fibers are well established.

Since the caudal edge of the putamen (419) of the lentiform nucleus has just appeared in the figure, the region labeled "retrolenticular internal capsule" in the previous sections is now labeled "posterior limb" (418). The sublenticular part of the posterior limb is present in the following section (445, Fig. 28).

Because both the lateral ventricle and the caudate nucleus are roughly C-shaped in the rostral-caudal plane, a transverse section will transect them twice. This figure shows the body (406) and the inferior horn (426) of the lateral ventricle. Similarly, the tail of the caudate nucleus (443) is labeled once in the floor of the body of the ventricle and again in the roof of the inferior horn.

The epithalamus is represented here by the habenular nuclei (315) and by the fasciculus retroflexus (318). This large tract takes its origin principally from the habenula and terminates in the interpeduncular nucleus (213, Fig. 28). Only the dorsal part of the fasciculus is distinct in this figure.

The figure shows the cistern of the great cerebral veins. This large subarachnoid space is bounded by the tela choroidea of the third ventricle (311), both pulvinars (324), the crura of the fornix (410), and the corpus callosum. The internal cerebral veins (452) are located centrally within the cistern.

10—Medial lemniscus
31—Ventral central trigeminal tract
133—Lateral spinothalamic tract
207—Oculomotor fibers
213—Interpeduncular nucleus
214—Red nucleus
219—Cerebellothalamic (dentato-thalamic) tract
220—Crus cerebri (pes pedunculi)
221—Substantia nigra
230—Rubrothalamic fibers
311—Tela choroidea of the third ventricle
315—Habenula
318—Fasciculus retroflexus
324—Pulvinar
330—Central (centromedian) nucleus
332—Posteromedial ventral nucleus of the thalamus
336—Posterolateral ventral nucleus of the thalamus
418—Posterior limb of the internal capsule
419—Putamen
433—Alveus
439—Dentate gyrus
443—Tail of the caudate nucleus
455—Vena and stria terminalis

27

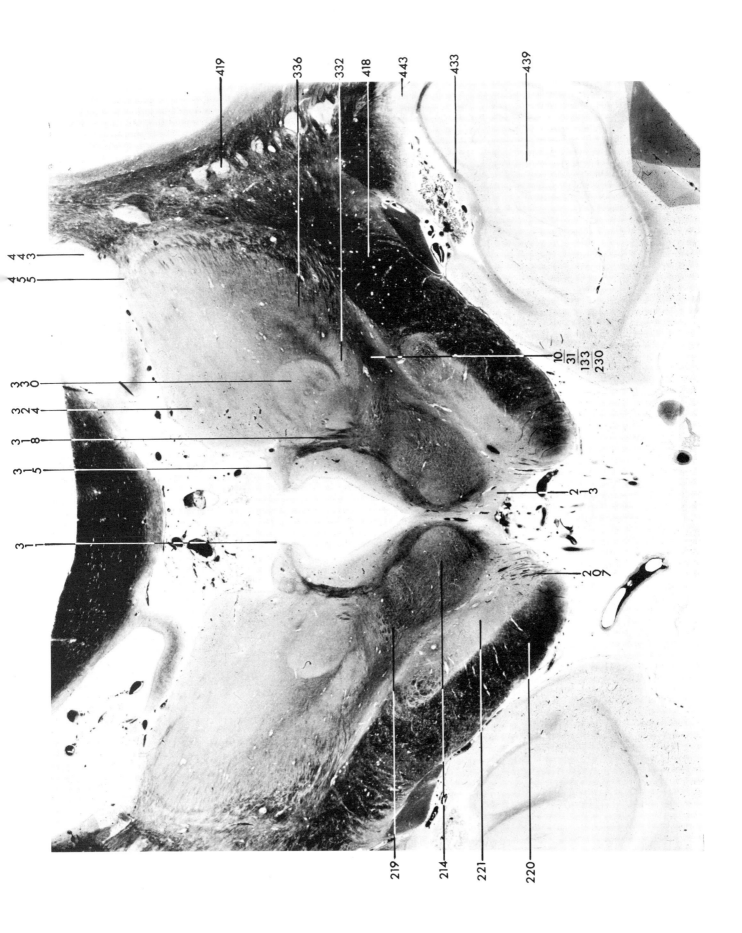

FIGURE 28. Caudal Thalamus

Superficially, Figure 28 is quite similar to the previous section. However, the habenula is now replaced by the fibers of the stria medullaris thalami (316) which extend caudally from their origin in the paraterminal gyrus (462) and the subcallosal area (463, Fig. 38), collectively the septal region, and in the anterior thalamic nucleus (326, Fig. 36) to synapse in the habenula (315, Fig. 27). The ventral part of the fasciculus retroflexus (318) is also included close to its synapse in the interpeduncular nuclei (213). Thus, several parts of a multineuronal chain between the septal area and the anterior thalamic and the interpeduncular nuclei are visible—stria medullaris, (habenula), fasciculus retroflexus, and interpeduncular nucleus.

The internal medullary lamina of the thalamus (339) is present as a thin line of myelinated fibers which separate the medial nucleus (317) from the several nuclei in the lateral mass of the thalamus. There are numerous small nuclei within the lamina, which are collectively denoted the intralaminar nuclei, but the only large intralaminar nucleus is the central (330). Rostrally the lamina splits to embrace the anterior nucleus (326, Fig. 36), but it is not considered an intralaminar nucleus. Other numerous but small nuclei are those of the midline (341), which occupy the periventricular gray matter adjacent to the third ventricle (307). The lateral mass of the thalamus here contains the posterior lateral nucleus (335) and the posterolateral ventral nucleus (336) and posteromedial ventral (332) nuclei.

The medial and posterior lateral nuclei are classified as associational nuclei, since their afferent connections are with other thalamic nuclei and with the cerebral cortex. Direct connections with the brain stem are lacking. The medial nucleus receives, principally, axons from other thalamic nuclei, from the hypothalamus, and from the frontal cerebral hemisphere ahead of the motor area. Efferent connections are with the same frontal cortex and with the hypothalamus. The posterior lateral nucleus has only afferent intrathalamic and parietal cortical connections. No precise functions are as yet known for this nucleus. Inferences, based upon the deficits resulting from cerebral cortical lesions, suggest that the medial nucleus may contribute drive and emotional overtones, through its hypothalamic connections, to the higher psychic functions of the prefrontal cortex. Lesions in the superior parietal area suggest that the posterior lateral thalamic nucleus contributes to the development of concepts of one's body. Both clearly have more complex functions than do such thalamic relay nuclei as the posteromedial ventral and posterolateral ventral nuclei (332 and 336), which receive the suprasegmental fibers of general sensation.

In the area of heavily myelinated fibers dorsolateral of the red nucleus (214), only the cerebellothalamic (219) and rubrothalamic (230) fibers are specifically labeled. Other ascending fibers are some lemniscal fibers which have not yet terminated in the posteromedial ventral (332) and posterolateral ventral (336) nuclei, and descending extrapyramidal fibers previously discussed in connection with Figure 25. Some other extrapyramidal fibers from the corpus striatum form a capsule along the dorsal and lateral edges of the subthalamic nucleus (331), which is just included in this section. These extrapyramidal fibers terminate in the subthalamus and in the substantia nigra (221).

Fibers to the substantia nigra originate principally from the caudate nucleus (443, Fig. 27) and the putamen (419, Fig. 30) and are called strionigral fibers. Those to the subthalamic nucleus are pallidosubthalamic fibers because they arise in the globus pallidus (421, Fig. 29).

Another subdivision of the posterior limb of the internal capsule is the sublenticular part (445), lying in the roof of the inferior horn of the lateral ventricle (426), ventral to the putamen (419) of the lentiform nucleus. Its name is derived from this relation. A major constituent of the sublenticular part is that portion of the geniculocalcarine tract which extends rostrally in the roof of the inferior horn before curving back, as the loop of Meyer and Archambault, to rejoin the rest of the geniculocalcarine tract. Auditory radiations also enter this subdivision to a slight extent, but most auditory fibers are in the retrolenticular part of the internal capsule. Corresponding corticifugal fibers to the lateral and medial geniculate nuclei probably accompany the optic and auditory radiations.

213—Interpeduncular nucleus
219—Cerebellothalamic (dentatothalamic) tract
230—Rubrothalamic fibers
307—Third ventricle
316—Stria medullaris of the thalamus
317—Medial (dorsal medial) nucleus of the thalamus
318—Fasciculus retroflexus
328—Optic tract
330—Central (centromedian) nucleus
331—Subthalamic nucleus
332—Posteromedial ventral nucleus of the thalamus
334—External medullary lamina of the thalamus
335—Posterior lateral nucleus of the thalamus
336—Posterolateral ventral nucleus of the thalamus
339—Internal medullary lamina of the thalamus
340—Reticular nuclei of the thalamus
341—Midline nuclei of the thalamus
406—Body of the lateral ventricle
408—Tela choroidea of the lateral ventricle
410—Crus of the fornix
419—Putamen
426—Inferior horn of the lateral ventricle
432—Hippocampus
433—Alveus
439—Dentate gyrus
445—Sublenticular part of the internal capsule
452—Inferior cerebral veins
454—Uncinate gyrus

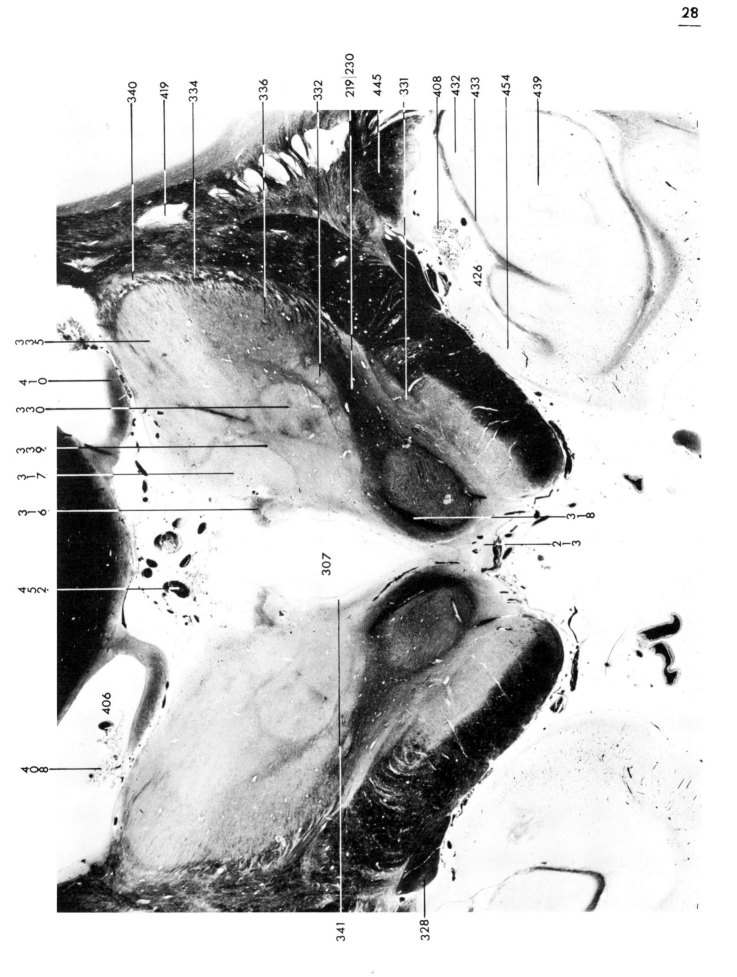

FIGURE 29. Caudal Thalamus and Hypothalamus

Figure 29 includes only the rostral tip of the substantia nigra (221), but a large area of the subthalamic nucleus (331) is present. Strionigral fibers form a slender lamina of myelinated fibers between the subthalamic nucleus and the substantia nigra. The mamillary bodies (300), the most caudal of the nuclei in the hypothalamus, are just making an appearance.

Lateral to the posterior limb of the internal capsule (418) are the globus pallidus (421) and the putamen (419), collectively called the lentiform nucleus. This nucleus lies medial to the insular cortex but is separated from it by the external (451) and extreme (456) capsules and the intervening nucleus, the claustrum (457). Fibers from the cerebral cortex enter the lentiform nucleus from both internal and external capsules. The external capsule is a possible pathway for impulses to the lentiform nucleus which could escape injury in lesions of the internal capsule. The extreme capsule is probably homologous to cerebral white matter.

The anterior choroidal artery (425) is labeled at two points on the *left*. The artery extends caudally along the ventral aspect of the optic tract (328). Multiple branches pierce the optic tract and vascularize it before entering to form a capillary bed in the globus pallidus (421) and the ventral part of the posterior limb of the internal capsule (418). On the *right*, such unlabeled branches of the anterior choroidal artery are visible as empty vessels in the medial part of the globus pallidus (421). The main vessel can be followed caudally, adjacent to and sending branches into the tela choroidea (408) of the inferior horn of the lateral ventricle (426, Figs. 28 to 26). A posterior choroidal branch of the posterior cerebral artery also vascularizes this choroid plexus of the inferior horn.

Only the rostral tip of the hippocampus still projects into the inferior horn of the lateral ventricle. Medial to it the cerebral gray matter is thickened because of the amygdaloid nucleus (427), which is covered by cortical gray matter of the uncus. The streaks of myelinated fibers in the lateral edge of the amygdala can be traced in more rostral sections into the anterior commissure (305, Figs. 31 to 33). An efferent tract of the amygdaloid nucleus is the stria terminalis (455). The major terminations of these fibers are in the anterior hypothalamus and preoptic area (Figs. 34, 35), paraterminal gyrus, and subcallosal area (462, 463, Fig. 38). But to reach these nuclei the stria follows a long devious course. The stria terminalis, also known as the stria semicircularis, the fornix, and the caudate have similar C-shaped configurations and are close together throughout much of their extent. The stria and tail of the caudate nucleus (443, Fig. 27) begin immediately caudal of the amygdaloid nucleus in the roof of the inferior horn; stria is always medial of the caudate nucleus. Just as the fimbria of the fornix (440) curves dorsally to become the crus of the fornix (410) in Figure 22, so also the stria (and the caudate nucleus) becomes recurrent and begins a course parallel with the terminal vein (455, Fig. 23), hence the similarity of names. Thereafter, both stria and vena terminalis lie in a groove between the thalamus and the caudate nucleus (443, Fig. 25) in the floor of the body of the lateral ventricle (406, Fig. 26) and can be followed rostrally as far as Figure 35. The stria then courses ventrally over the rostral curvature of the thalamus to reach the terminations mentioned above. Thus, this fiber tract connects the lateral part (amygdaloid nucleus) of the limbic system with the medial part (subcallosal area and paraterminal gyrus). The stria is primarily an efferent tract of the amygdaloid nucleus, but it may also contain afferent fibers. The nucleus is known to receive fibers from the lateral olfactory stria. The results of extirpation and stimulation of the amygdaloid nucleus indicate that it affects behavior and *visceral* responses mediated by the involuntary nervous system. In this relation the anatomic connection of the stria terminalis with the hypothalamus is suggestive.

The terminal vein (455), which largely parallels the stria terminalis in the floor of the body of the lateral ventricle, drains blood from the caudate and lentiform nuclei, the thalamus, and parts of the internal capsule into the internal cerebral veins (452).

202—Posteromedial striate arteries
214—Red nucleus
219—Cerebellothalamic (dentato-thalamic) tract
221—Substantia nigra
230—Rubrothalamic fibers
300—Mamillary nucleus
311—Tela choroidea of the third ventricle
331—Subthalamic nucleus
335—Posterior lateral nucleus of the thalamus
341—Midline nuclei of the thalamus
410—Crus of the fornix
411—Tegmental area H
418—Posterior limb of the internal capsule
421—Globus pallidus
425—Anterior choroidal artery
427—Amygdaloid nucleus
432—Hippocampus
451—External capsule
452—Internal cerebral veins
455—Vena and stria terminalis
456—Extreme capsule
457—Claustrum

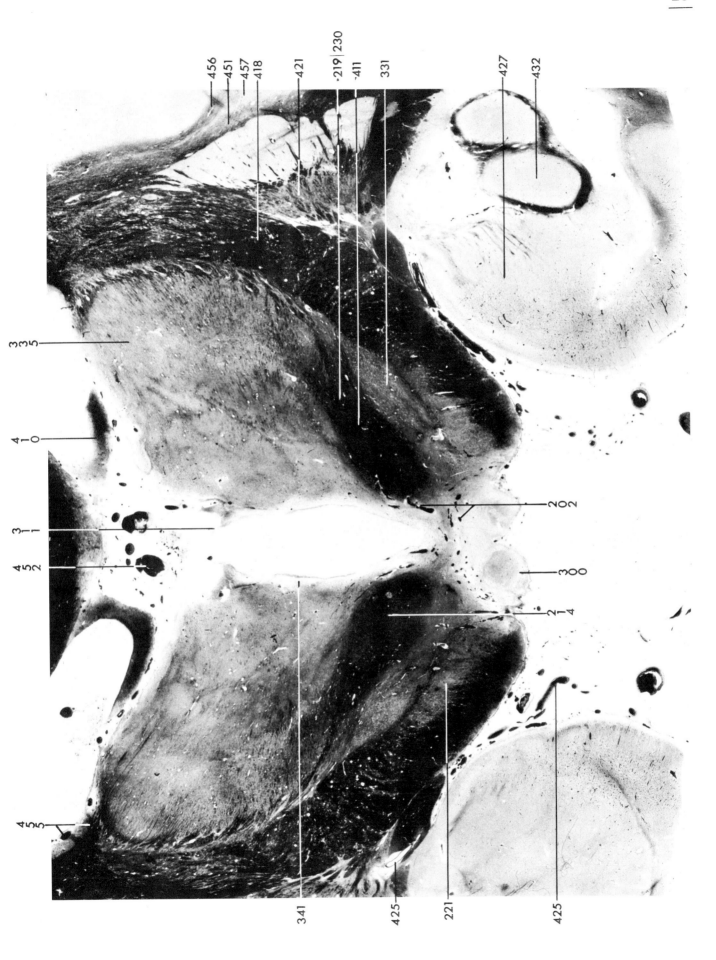

FIGURE 30. Midthalamus

The four major divisions of the diencephalon are all included in Figure 30. A line drawn from each hypothalamic sulcus (342) (not very distinct in this brain) to the medial edge of each crus cerebri (220) delimits the hypothalamus (343) (between the two lines) from the rest of the diencephalon. In three dimensions the hypothalamus resembles a prism. The subthalamus lies lateral to the hypothalamus in the ventral part of the diencephalon; besides the prominent subthalamic nucleus (331) it includes tegmental areas H (411), H_1 (414), and H_2 (412) and the zona incerta (415). The epithalamus is here represented only by the stria medullaris thalami (316). Further caudal, the habenula (315, Fig. 27) and the pineal body (308, Fig. 23) also are parts of the epithalamus. The rest of the diencephalon is the dorsal thalamus, or thalamus proper. In it, at this level, the large medial nucleus (317) is separated from the lateral thalamic nuclei by the internal medullary lamina (339). Of these lateral nuclei, the section still includes, dorsally, the posterior lateral nucleus (335). Ventrally, however, the intermediate ventral nucleus (337) now occupies the same relative position as did the two posterior ventral nuclei (332 and 336, Fig. 28). Cerebellothalamic fibers terminate largely in the intermediate and anterior ventral nuclei. They are thalamic relay nuclei, since they project axons conveying impulses from the cerebellum to the motor areas in the frontal lobe, rostral of the central sulcus. These corticicipetal axons and the reciprocal corticothalamic fibers to the intermediate ventral nucleus (340) as they course through it to enter or leave the posterior limb of the internal capsule (418).

The three tegmental areas (411, 412, and 414) are largely occupied by axons whose cell bodies are located chiefly in the globus pallidus (421) of the lentiform nucleus. These axons either pass through the internal capsule as the fasciculus lenticularis (459, Figs. 33 to 31) or pass around its rostral edge as the ansa lenticularis (413, Figs. 35 to 31) to accumulate in tegmental area H_2 (412). A smaller part of the fibers in the area H_2 continues a caudal course to synapse in prerubral nuclei in area H (411) or descend among the fibers along the ventrolateral side of the red nucleus (214, Figs. 29 to 25) to synapse in the pedunculopontine nucleus (see comment on Figs. 21 and 22). Most axons enter tegmental area H_2 rostral to the present plane, so H_2 is very slender here. As they course caudally, the fibers shift medially and so come to occupy tegmental area H (411), sometimes called the prerubral field. Some pallidal efferent fibers traverse the internal capsule and synapse in the subthalamic nucleus without entering H_2. Strionigral fibers (453, Fig. 25) from the putamen (419) also do not enter H_2.

Most of the axons in tegmental area H become recurrent, ascend rostrally in tegmental area H_1 (414), and synapse in the intermediate ventral nucleus (337) and in the anterior ventral nucleus (329, Fig. 36). Fibers also terminate in the central nucleus (330, Fig. 28). Hence, tegmental area H_1 is also called the thalamic fasciculus. Cerebellothalamic fibers (219) are also a component of the fasciculus. Both anterior ventral and intermediate ventral nuclei project axons, via the internal capsule, to the precentral and adjacent motor gyri in the frontal cortex. Since the corpus striatum receives axons of cerebral cortical neurons, the globus pallidus and its ascending axons in tegmental area H_1 are thought to function as part of a feedback circuit, modulating the efferent outflow of impulses in pyramidal and cortically originating extrapyramidal fiber tracts to motor nuclei in the brain stem and spinal cord, and to the cerebellum, via olivocerebellar and pontocerebellar fibers.

The mamillary nuclei have two prominent fiber connections. The one visible here is the mamillothalamic fasciculus (313). This fasciculus courses dorsally and rostrally and connects, reciprocally, the anterior thalamic (326, Fig. 36) and the mamillary nuclei. It is a prominent fiber tract in all the intervening sections. Since the anterior nucleus is also reciprocally connected with the gyrus cinguli, the possibility exists that the cerebral cortex can modulate the activity of the mamillary nucleus and be modulated by it. It is instructive to see the mamillothalamic fasciculus in parasagittal Figures 50 to 52. The fornix is the other prominent fiber tract of the mamillary nucleus (403, Fig. 32).

220—Crus cerebri (pes pedunculi)
300—Mamillary nucleus
307—Third ventricle
313—Mamillothalamic fasciculus
316—Stria medullaris of the thalamus
317—Medial (dorsal medial) nucleus of the thalamus
328—Optic tract
331—Subthalamic nucleus
334—External medullary lamina of the thalamus
335—Posterior lateral nucleus of the thalamus
337—Intermediate ventral nucleus of the thalamus (VL)
339—Internal medullary lamina of the thalamus
340—Reticular nuclei of the thalamus
341—Midline nuclei of the thalamus
342—Hypothalamic sulcus
343—Hypothalamus
406—Body of the lateral ventricle
408—Tela choroidea of the lateral ventricle
411—Tegmental area H
412—Tegmental area H_2
414—Tegmental area H_1
415—Zona incerta
416—Internal carotid artery
419—Putamen
426—Inferior horn of the lateral ventricle
445—Sublenticular part of the internal capsule
454—Uncinate gyrus
458—Cortex of the insula

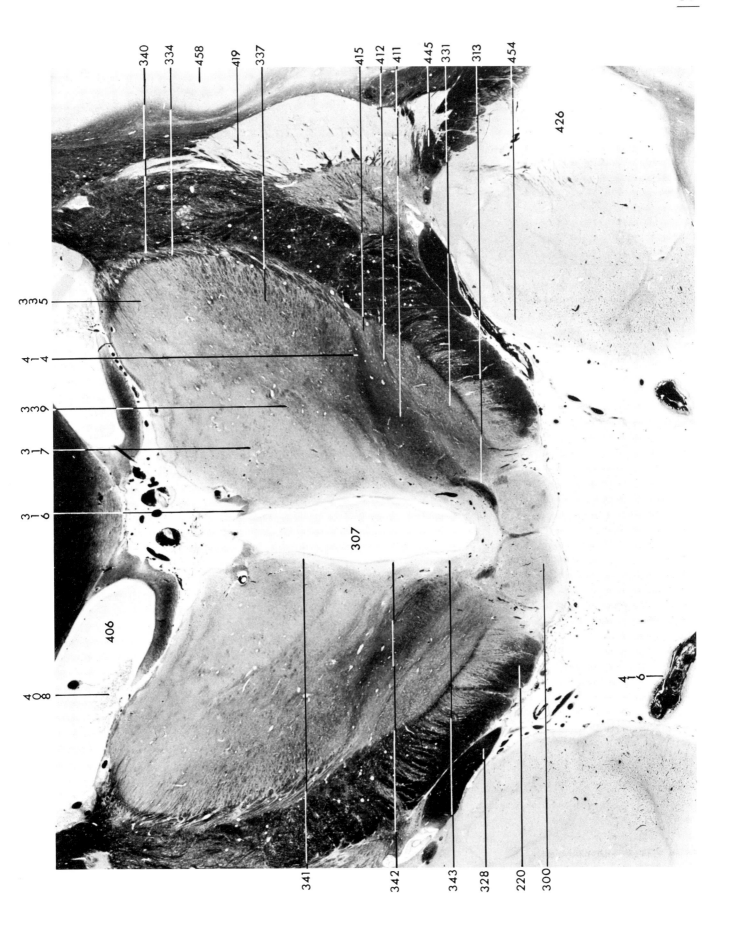

FIGURE 31. Midthalamus and the Tegmental Fields

Two major efferent tracts from the globus pallidus (421) are well shown. On the left side, myelinated fibers of the fascicularis lenticularis (459) can be followed from the medial division of the globus pallidus directly through the internal capsule (418) into tegmental area H₂ (412). The second group of issuing fibers forms the ansa lenticularis (413). This tract lies ventral to the globus pallidus and is continuous with the internal medullary lamina within the globus pallidus (429). Since fibers of the ansa lenticularis enter tegmental area H₂ by sweeping around the rostral edge of the internal capsule, this can only be visualized by following the ansa into more rostral Figures 34 and 35. The ansa can be thought of as a group of fibers similar in origin and destination to those which go directly through the internal capsule, but which have been displaced rostrally with the development of the internal capsule. Pallidosubthalamic and strionigral fibers follow independent courses through the internal capsule and do not traverse either H₂ or the ansa lenticularis.

Afferent fibers to the globus pallidus form tracts that are not visible in Weigert slides. Most areas of the cerebral cortex project axons to the caudate and putamen. These two nuclei in turn project fibers to the globus pallidus.

The efferent mamillothalamic fasciculus (313) begins as a capsule of myelinated fibers about the medial and rostral surfaces of the mamillary nucleus (300) before coursing dorsally along the medial side of tegmental area H (411). Its further course is seen in Figures 32 to 36. In contrast, the fibers from the hippocampus that form the column of the fornix (403, Fig. 32) enter the lateral side of the mamillary nucleus without forming a capsule. The continuity between the column (403) and the body (401) of the fornix can be verified by following them in Figures 32 to 36. A look at the body and column in sagittal figures 46 to 43 is beneficial.

The floor of the third ventricle (307) here is the tuber cinereum (344). This area of the hypothalamus is covered with the primary plexus of hypophyseal portal veins which supply blood to the pars distalis of the hypophysis. Axons of neurons, whose cell bodies form a series of nuclei in the tuber cinereum, terminate in relation to this primary plexus and release hormones into it that facilitate or inhibit the release of trophic hormones from cells of the pars distalis of the hypophysis.

The plane of section passes just rostral to the tip of the inferior horn of the lateral ventricle, and therefore includes a large section of the amygdaloid nucleus (427). Fibers (305) along its lateral edge can be followed into the anterior commissure in Figures 32 and 33.

300—Mamillary nucleus
305—Anterior commissure
311—Tela choroidea of the third ventricle
313—Mamillothalamic fasciculus
331—Subthalamic nucleus
337—Intermediate ventral nucleus of the thalamus
341—Midline nuclei of the thalamus
342—Hypothalamic sulcus
343—Hypothalamus
344—Tuber cinereum
402—Body of the corpus callosum
411—Tegmental area H
412—Tegmental area H₂
413—Ansa lenticularis
414—Tegmental area H₁
415—Zona incerta
416—Internal carotid artery
418—Posterior limb of the internal capsule
421—Globus pallidus
427—Amygdaloid nucleus
429—Internal medullary lamina of the globus pallidus
435—Body of the caudate nucleus
451—External capsule
455—Vena and stria terminalis
456—Extreme capsule
457—Claustrum
459—Fasciculus lenticularis

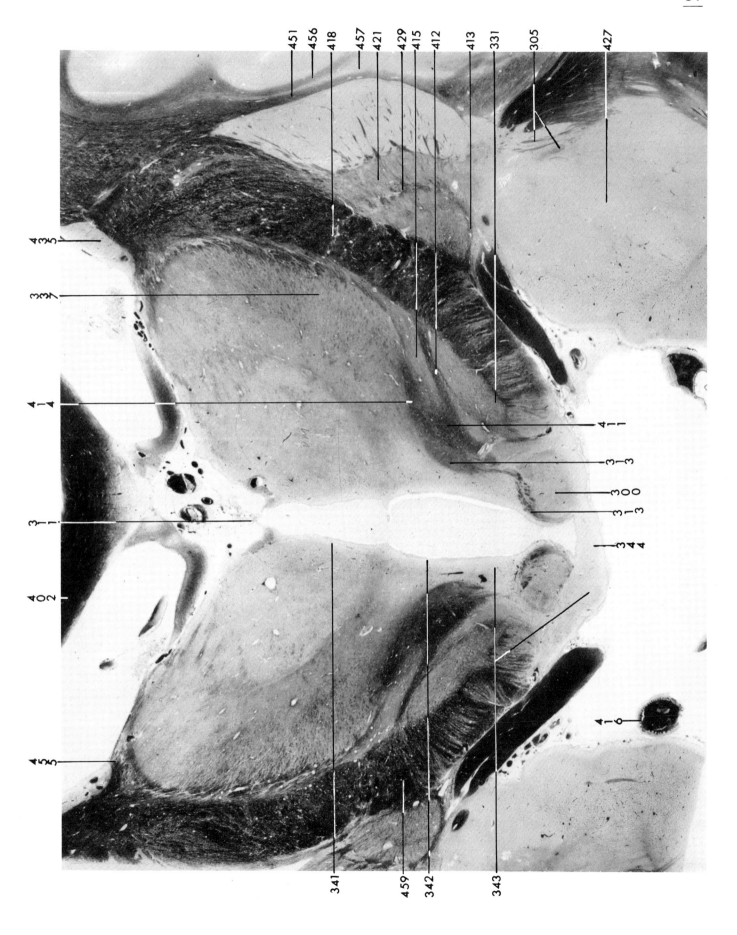

FIGURE 32.   Midthalamus and Interthalamic Adhesion

Figure 32 is included primarily to facilitate following the course of the mamillothalamic fasciculus and fibers in the column of the fornix. The mamillothalamic fasciculus (313) extends from the origin, obvious in its name (300, Fig. 30), to its major termination in the anterior nucleus of the thalamus (326, Fig. 36). This fasciculus not only extends rostrally but also dorsally, and therefore is progressively more dorsal in the intervening figures. The column of the fornix (403) follows a similar course rostrally through the hypothalamus toward its juncture with the body of the fornix (401) in Figure 38; it also is progressively more dorsal in the figures, but is always ventral to the mamillothalamic fasciculus.

The course of axons from the globus pallidus, which, as the fasciculus lenticularis (459, left side), pass directly through the internal capsule (418) to enter tegmental area H₂ (412), is readily followed. Dorsal to the tegmental fields, fibers which reciprocally connect the intermediate ventral nucleus (337) and the motor area of the frontal cortex obscure the reticular nucleus (340) as they pass through it, to, or from the internal capsule (418).

A strand of gray matter extends dorsally from the putamen (419) toward the body of the caudate nucleus (435). Putamen and caudate are actually one nuclear mass, partially separated by fibers of the internal capsule which traverse it. This is the basis for statements that the anterior limb of the internal capsule is part of the corpus striatum. In fact, only the gray matter is part of the corpus striatum.

Ventrally, the forked hypothalamic *leader* (343) terminates in the two major subdivisions of the hypothalamus, medial and lateral to the column of the fornix (403), which roughly subdivides the hypothalamus. On the *left*, the plane of section passes through the column

of the fornix and the medial mamillothalamic fasciculus (313) just rostral of the mamillary nucleus. On the *right*, the plane of section passes through the mamillary nucleus. The mamillothalamic fasciculus forms a capsule about the medial and dorsal curvature of the mamillary nucleus. Pale fibers within the nucleus, laterally, become the column of the fornix (403).

All of the midline and most of the other hypothalamic nuclei are located in the medial part of the hypothalamus; most of the fibers which course to, from, or through the hypothalamus occupy the lateral hypothalamus. One such group of fibers, the medial forebrain bundle, occupies the lightly stained area immediately lateral to the mamillary nucleus (300). At this level the bundle contains, among others, ascending fibers from reticular neurons of the brain stem and descending fibers from various hypothalamic nuclei to reticular and visceral motor nerve nuclei. Precise anatomical data are not available.

Tuberal nuclei begin to occupy the superficial aspect of both the medial and the lateral divisions of the hypothalamus just rostral to the plane of this section. It is the hormones from these tuberal nuclei which enter the hypophyseal portal circulation on the tuber cinereum (344) and modulate secretory activity of the anterior pituitary cells.

300—Mamillary nucleus
305—Anterior commissure
307—Third ventricle
313—Mamillothalamic fasciculus
316—Stria medullaris of the thalamus
317—Medial (dorsal medial) nucleus of the thalamus
328—Optic tract
331—Subthalamic nucleus
334—External medullary lamina of the thalamus
337—Intermediate ventral nucleus of the thalamus
339—Internal medullary lamina of the thalamus
340—Reticular nuclei of the thalamus
341—Midline nuclei of the thalamus
342—Hypothalamic sulcus
343—Hypothalamus
344—Tuber cinereum
345—Interthalamic adhesion (massa intermedia)
401—Body of the fornix
403—Column of the fornix
406—Body of the lateral ventricle
408—Tela choroidea of the lateral ventricle
411—Tegmental area H
412—Tegmental area H₂
414—Tegmental area H₁
415—Zona incerta
416—Internal carotid artery
419—Putamen
452—Internal cerebral veins
454—Uncinate gyrus
459—Fascicularis lenticularis

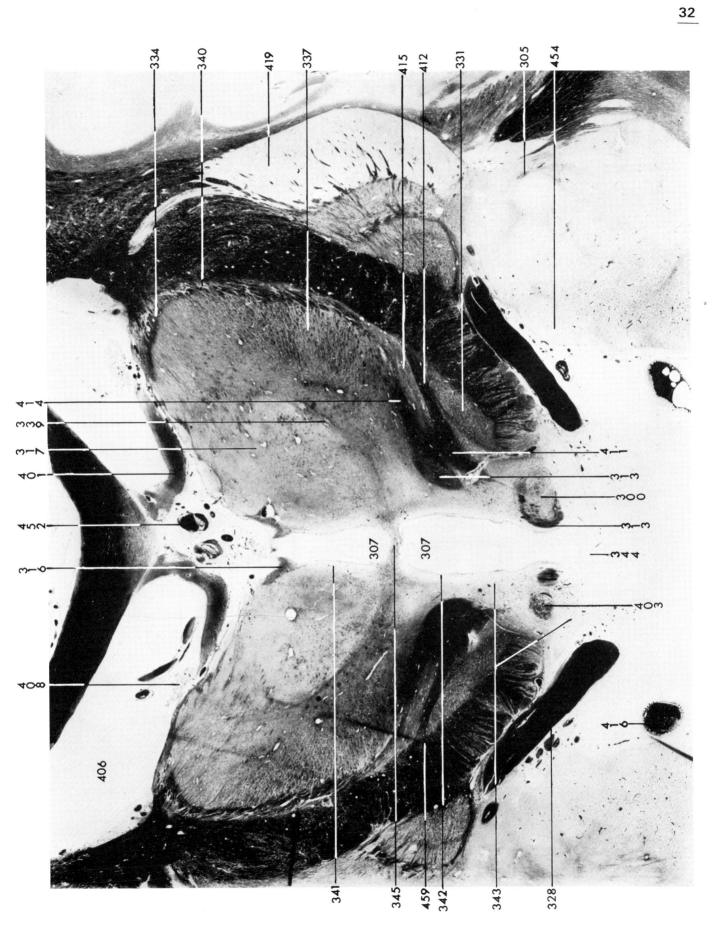

FIGURE 33.

Midthalamus at Junction of Optic Nerve and Tract

The cross-sectional area of the hypothalamus is maximal in Figure 33. The columns of the fornix (403), which are cut almost in cross sections as they course caudally toward the mamillary nuclei, occupy a more dorsal position in the hypothalamus (343). It is instructive to see the columns in Figure 46, a sagittal section. Ventrally the infundibular stalk (301) of the neurohypophysis takes off from the tuber cinereum (344), which is here covered by the primary vascular plexus of the hypophyseal portal system. The infundibular stalk contains the axons of the supraoptic and paraventricular nuclei, which extend into the infundibular process of the neurohypophysis. The supraoptic nucleus occupies both lateral and medial hypothalamus, where it sits astride the optic tracts (328) and optic chiasm (302, Fig. 34). The paraventricular nucleus is situated in the medial hypothalamus approximately where the *upper* hypothalamic *leader* (343) terminates. These two nuclei secrete the hormones, oxytocin and vasopressin, stored in, and released from, the neurohypophysis.

The section of the mamillothalamic fasciculus (313) has shifted dorsally away from tegmental area H_1 (414), and lies in the ventral and medial edge of the intermediate ventral nucleus (337). The dorsal lateral nucleus (325) is obvious now as an elliptic mass separated on its ventral aspect by myelinated fibers from the dorsal medial (317) and intermediate ventral (337) nuclei. In Figures 32 to 29, where it is unlabeled, the dorsal lateral nucleus is smaller, and the myelinated fibers which delimit it are fewer and less well stained. Caudally it blends with the pulvinar. The length of this nucleus is better appreciated in Figures 46 to 49. Because it has connections with the gyrus cinguli, it is sometimes regarded as a caudal extension of the anterior nucleus (326, Fig. 36). Its function is obscure.

On the *left side*, the ansa lenticularis (413) is just beginning to sweep around the internal capsule to become incorporated in tegmental area H_2 (412). The ansa appears to pass ventral to the internal capsule here only because its rostral edge is oblique with reference to the dorsal-ventral axis of the cerebrum. Many more fibers, issuing from the lentiform nucleus, traverse the internal capsule in the fasciculus lenticularis (459) and enter tegmental area H_2. Tegmental area H_1 (414) is reduced in size, since many pallidothalamic fibers have already synapsed in the intermediate ventral nucleus (337) caudal to this level. Tegmental area H is wholly caudal. Visible here, on the *right side* particularly, a few tegmental fibers arch over the column of the fornix and enter the medial hypothalamus. Although they are frequently designated "pallidohypothalamic," it is questionable whether these fibers do synapse in the hypothalamus. They may be recurrent pallidothalamic fibers.

The fibers which constitute the anterior commissure (305) are now a distinct bundle ventral to the putamen (419). This commissure is a prominent tract in all the remaining transverse figures.

The internal carotid artery (416), which was present in Figures 30 to 32, is here bifurcating into the anterior cerebral artery (404) and the middle cerebral artery (428, Fig. 34). The small vessels in the subarachnoid space dorsal to the anterior cerebral artery are anteromedial branches of it and anterolateral striate branches of the middle cerebral artery. These small vessels penetrate the triangular area of cerebrum ventral to the ansa lenticularis (413) called the anterior perforated substance. Upon extending dorsally they vascularize the lateral part of the lentiform nucleus and the dorsal part of the internal capsule. As previously noted (Fig. 29),

the medial part of the lentiform nucleus and the ventral part of the internal capsule receive blood from branches of the anterior choroidal artery.

301—Infundibular stalk
305—Anterior commissure
307—Third ventricle
311—Tela choroidea of the third ventricle
313—Mamillothalamic fasciculus
325—Dorsal lateral nucleus of the thalamus
337—Intermediate ventral nucleus of the thalamus
341—Midline nuclei of the thalamus
342—Hypothalamic sulcus
343—Hypothalamus
344—Tuber cinereum
345—Interthalamic adhesion (massa intermedia)
402—Body of the corpus callosum
403—Column of the fornix
404—Anterior cerebral artery
408—Tela choroidea of the lateral ventricle
412—Tegmental area H_2
413—Ansa lenticularis
414—Tegmental area H_1
415—Zona incerta
418—Posterior limb of the internal capsule
421—Globus pallidus
427—Amygdaloid nucleus
435—Body of the caudate nucleus
451—External capsule
452—Internal capsule
455—Vena and stria terminalis
457—Claustrum
459—Fasciculus lenticularis

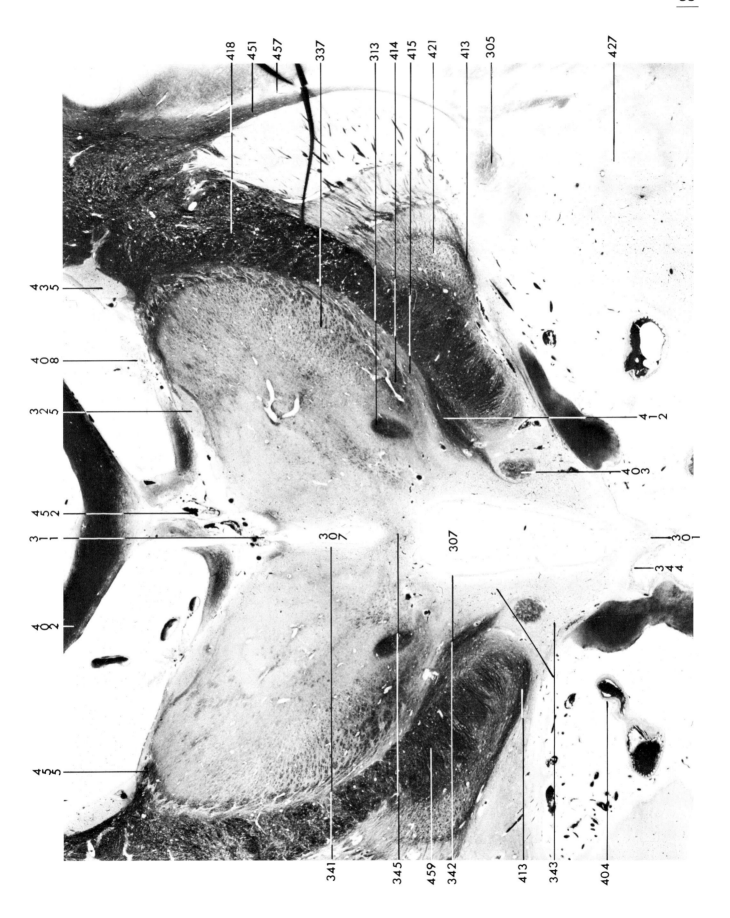

FIGURE 34. Optic Chiasm and Rostral Thalamus

The cardinal features here are the optic chiasm (302), where axons arising in nasal retinal quadrants cross, the optic nerve (314), and the optic tract (328). The slender fiber tract (unlabeled, *right side*) slightly detached from the optic tracts is part of the dorsal supraoptic decussation (Meynert's). It contains crossing fibers from the subthalamic nucleus to the globus pallidus.

Medial and in part ventral to the mamillothalamic fasciculus (313) is the inferior thalamic peduncle (460). The *leader* terminates in the most compact part of the fasciculus, but obliquely sectioned fibers can be followed dorsally to the medial nucleus (317). Neither the composition nor the function of the inferior peduncle is well established. Many of its fibers connect the thalamus—chiefly its medial nucleus—with the hypothalamus (343), amygdaloid nucleus (427), and orbital cerebral cortex. The physical possibility for these cortical, lentiform, and amygdaloid connections can be visualized if inferior thalamic peduncle (460) is followed into Figure 35. Access to the hypothalamus is obvious here. That part of the fibers in the peduncle which connect the prefrontal cortex and hypothalamus via an intermediate synapse in the medial nucleus may contribute a cast of emotion or feeling overtone to the higher psychic functions of the prefrontal cortex and therefore may affect personality.

On the *right side* of the figure one of the anterolateral striate arteries (434) can be followed through the anterior perforated substance (461) into the internal medullary lamina of the globus pallidus (429) toward the dorsal part of the posterior limb of the internal capsule (418). All of these regions named are vascularized by anterolateral striate arteries. Cerebrovascular accidents involving these vessels produce deficits which are a result of interruption in conduction of impulses by the fibers constituting the internal

capsule. At this level in the posterior limb of the internal capsule (418) these would include fibers from and to the posteromedial and posterolateral thalamic radiation (including fibers from and to the posteromedial and posterolateral ventral nuclei (332 and 336, Fig. 28) and the postcentral gyrus), corticospinal, corticopontine, corticoreticular, and corticorubral fibers. Corticospinal fibers affecting the upper extremity lie closer to the genu of the internal capsule (422, Fig. 37) than those to the trunk, which are rostral to those affecting the leg. The most obvious effects of a stroke are, therefore, paralysis of volitional movements and sensory deficits. The location of the cortical fibers to the lentiform, subthalamic, and substantia nigra nuclei are not established anatomically, but it is conceivable that they also are in the posterior limb.

The ansa lenticularis (413) has been labeled twice on the *left* and once on the *right* to mark the course of these fibers around the rostral edge of the internal capsule so as to enter tegmental field H₂ (412, Fig. 33). All of the fibers in the thalamic fasciculus which have been coursing through tegmental area H₁ either have now synapsed in the intermediate ventral nucleus (337) or are traversing its ventral aspect to reach the anterior ventral nucleus (329, Fig. 36).

The uncinate fasciculus (unlabeled) occupies the large myelinated area ventral to the claustrum (457) and lateral to the amygdaloid nucleus (427). This long associational bundle connects the orbital and inferior parts of the frontal cortex with the rostral part of the temporal lobe.

302—Optic chiasm
307—Third ventricle
313—Mamillothalamic fasciculus
314—Optic nerve
316—Stria medullaris of the thalamus
317—Medial (dorsal medial) nucleus of the thalamus
325—Dorsal lateral nucleus of the thalamus
328—Optic tract
334—External medullary lamina of the thalamus
337—Intermediate ventral nucleus of the thalamus
339—Internal medullary lamina of the thalamus
341—Midline nuclei of the thalamus
342—Hypothalamic sulcus
343—Hypothalamus
401—Body of the fornix
404—Anterior cerebral artery
406—Body of the lateral ventricle
413—Ansa lenticularis
419—Putamen
428—Middle cerebral artery
429—Internal medullary lamina of the globus pallidus
434—Anterolateral striate branches of the middle cerebral artery
451—External capsule
452—Internal cerebral veins
456—Extreme capsule
460—Inferior thalamic peduncle

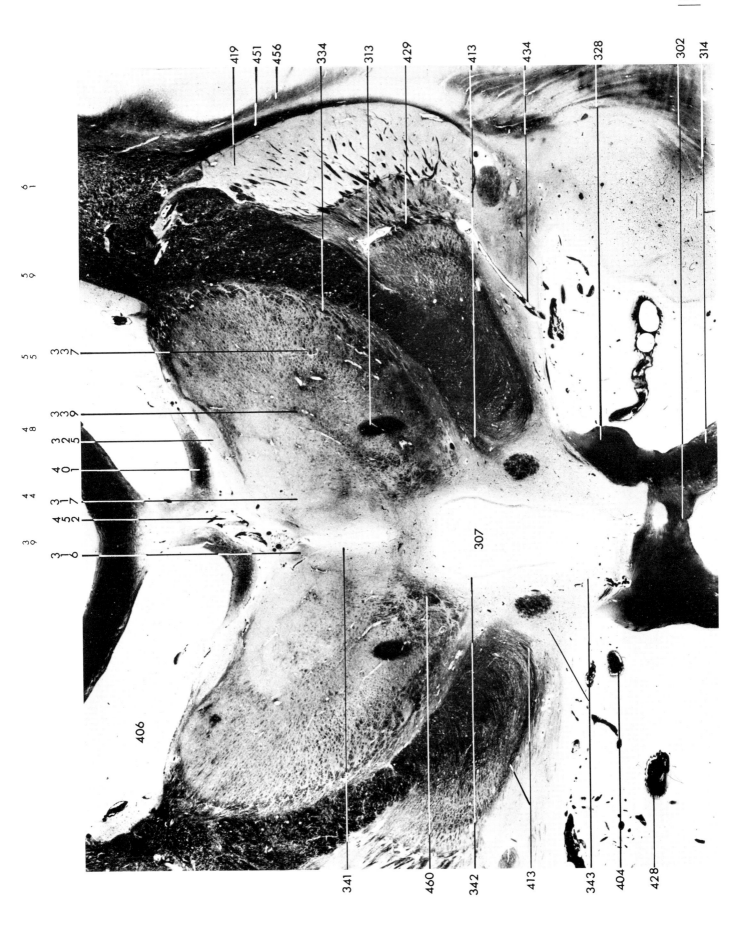

FIGURE 35.

Optic Chiasm, Rostral Thalamus, and Hypothalamus

The plane of Figure 35 passes through the rostral ends of the medial nucleus (317), intermediate ventral nucleus (337), interthalamic adhesion (345), optic chiasm (302), and amygdaloid nucleus (427); hence these structures are not included in the following sections. The position of the mamillothalamic tract (313) has shifted still further dorsal toward its chief termination in the anterior thalamic nucleus (326, Fig. 36). The column of the fornix (403) also is shifted closer to its continuity with the body of the fornix (401, Fig. 38). Sweeping around the rostral edge of the internal capsule (418) is the ansa lenticularis (413). Ventral of the ansa lenticularis, fibers of the ansa peduncularis extend through the anterior perforated substance (461). Some curve dorsally around the internal capsule and enter the thalamus as the inferior thalamic peduncle (460). Other fibers (unstained) of the ansa peduncularis continue medially into the hypothalamus. The inferior thalamic peduncle reciprocally connects the medial nucleus (317) with the amygdaloid nucleus (427), temporal, and orbitofrontal cortices. The unstained fibers of the ansa extend between the hypothalamus and the temporal, orbitofrontal cortices.

In transverse sections the transition between anterior (423) and posterior (418) limbs of the internal capsule is not obvious as it is in a horizontal section. The anterior limb, however, lies between the caudate nucleus (435) and the putamen (419). These two nuclei are joined together by gray matter extending into the anterior internal capsule, as can be seen here. The posterior limb (418) is situated between the thalamus and the lentiform nucleus. Here it is beginning to diminish in size as its rostral extent is approached.

Turning to arteries, the anterior cerebral (404) itself is adjacent to the hypothalamus ventrally, while the small, unlabeled cortical

vessels dorsal to the corpus callosum (402) are branches of it. To reach this dorsal position, the anterior cerebral artery curves around the rostral end of the diencephalon and the corpus callosum. The cortical branches are distributed primarily on the medial surfaces of the frontal and parietal lobes as far caudally as the occipital lobe, and to orbitofrontal cortex.

The middle cerebral artery (428) is the other terminal branch of the internal carotid. It runs laterally, giving off many anterolateral striate vessels (434) which enter the anterior perforated substance (461) and vascularize the lentiform nucleus and the dorsal part of the internal capsule, as previously noted. The main artery extends laterally and passes through the lateral fissure of Sylvius (428, Figs. 36 and 37) to emerge on the lateral cerebral surface. Its branches supply almost the entire lateral aspects of the frontal, parietal, temporal, and occipital lobes. However, the anterior cerebral artery extends onto the lateral aspects of the frontal and parietal lobes to a slight extent; the posterior cerebral artery covers the medial surface of the occipital lobe (see legend of Fig. 22 (407) and Figs. 44 to 52) and the inferior surface of the temporal lobe; it extends to a degree onto their lateral aspects.

302—Optic chiasm
305—Anterior commissure
313—Mamillothalamic fasciculus
325—Dorsal lateral nucleus of the thalamus
337—Intermediate ventral nucleus of the thalamus
340—Reticular nucleus of the thalamus
341—Midline nuclei of the thalamus
342—Hypothalamic sulcus
345—Interthalamic adhesion (massa intermedia)
402—Body of the corpus callosum
403—Column of the fornix
404—Anterior cerebral artery
408—Tela choroidea of the lateral ventricle
413—Ansa lenticularis
418—Posterior limb of the internal capsule
421—Globus pallidus
423—Anterior limb of the internal capsule
427—Amygdaloid nucleus
428—Middle cerebral artery
434—Anterolateral striate branches of the middle cerebral artery
435—Body of the caudate nucleus
452—Internal cerebral veins
455—Vena and stria terminalis
460—Inferior thalamic peduncle
461—Anterior perforated substance

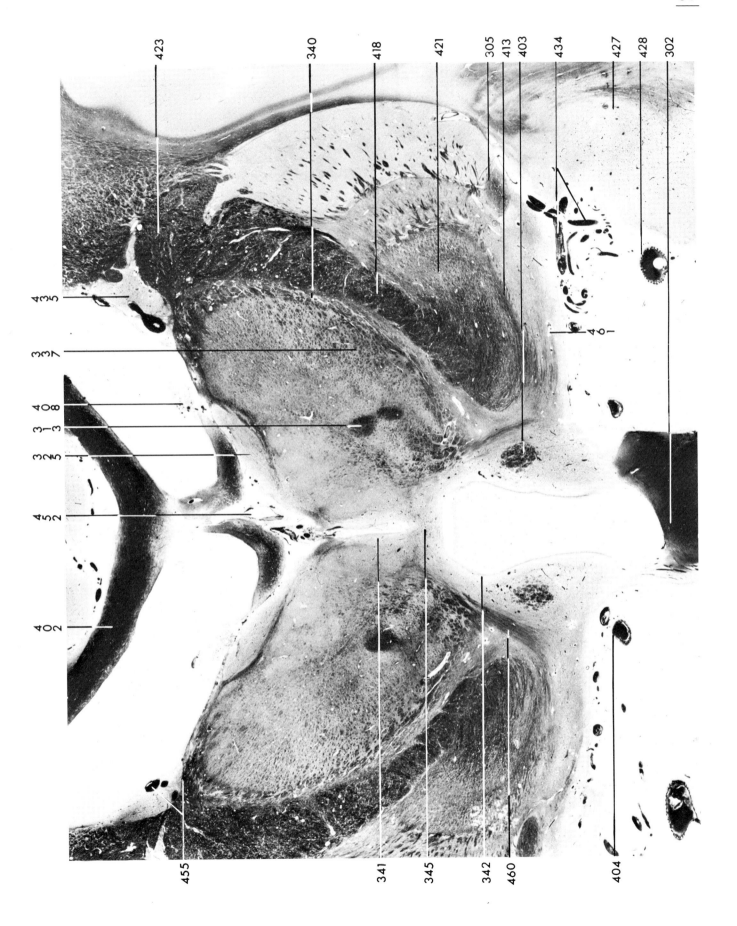

FIGURE 36.

Rostral Thalamus and Preoptic Hypothalamus

The plane of the figure includes a preoptic segment of the hypothalamus ventral to the column of the fornix (403), and the anterior (326) and anterior ventral (329) nuclei of the dorsal thalamus. The anterior ventral nucleus receives fibers from the globus pallidus and cerebellum via the thalamic fasciculus (H_1), from the cerebral cortex, and from the substantia nigra. There are two cytologically distinct subdivisions of the nucleus and some afferents do not synapse in both parts. The substantia nigra projects fibers only to the medial part, for example. The mamillothalamic fasciculus (313) is spread out as its fibers terminate in the anterior nucleus. Efferent connections of the anterior nucleus are with the gyrus cinguli and mamillary nucleus. Also some fibers enter the stria medullaris of the thalamus (316), and terminate in the habenular nucleus (315, Fig. 26). Other fibers in the stria medullaris originate in the subcallosal area and paraterminal gyrus (463 and 462, Figs. 38 and 37), collectively the septal area, and in the hippocampus. From the habenula, a pathway extends to motor nuclei in the brain stem and cord via the fasciculus retroflexus and the interpeduncular nucleus, as already outlined in connection with Figure 26. The exact function of this intricate, multineuronal pathway which arises in medial and lateral parts of the limbic system is not known. It may be an olfactory reflex path, in part.

On the *right side*, particularly, the inferior thalamic peduncle (460) appears to be entering the anterior ventral nucleus. The thin lamina terminalis (304) marks the rostral end of the prosencephalon in the midline. A more medial portion of the posterior forceps of the anterior commissure (305) is now included in the figure, ventral to the globus pallidus.

The middle cerebral artery (428) is sectioned in the lateral fissure of Sylvius in its passage to the lateral surface of the cerebrum.

304—Lamina terminalis
307—Third ventricle
311—Tela choroidea of the third ventricle
313—Mamillothalamic fasciculus
316—Stria medullaris of the thalamus
326—Anterior nucleus of the thalamus
329—Anterior ventral nucleus of the thalamus
342—Hypothalamic sulcus
401—Body of the fornix
404—Anterior cerebral artery
406—Body of the lateral ventricle
419—Putamen
423—Anterior limb of the internal capsule
428—Middle cerebral artery
429—Internal medullary lamina of the globus pallidus
451—External capsule
456—Extreme capsule
457—Claustrum
461—Anterior perforated substance

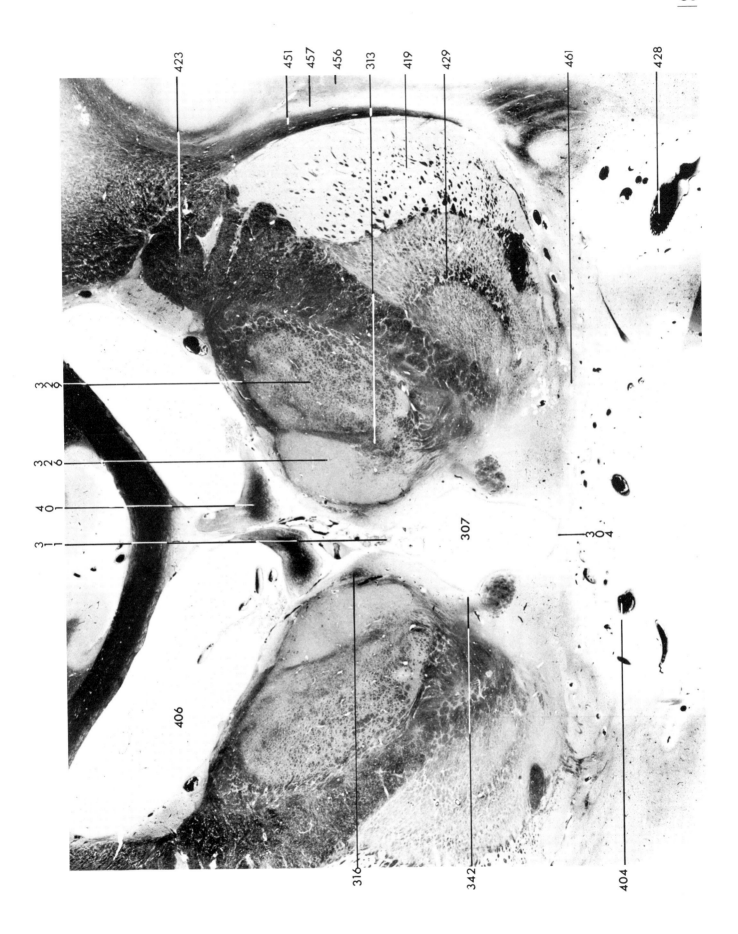

423

451
457
456

313

419

429

461

428

3 2 6

3 2 6

4 0

3 1

307

3 0 4

406

316

342

404

FIGURE 37.

Rostral Thalamus and Decussation of the Anterior Commissure

In Figure 37 the anterior commissure (305) sweeps across the section and actually decussates in the lamina terminalis (304, Fig. 36). On the *left*, the commissure bifurcates into a compact bundle and a diffuse group of fibers beneath the bundle. The compact fibers form the posterior forceps of the anterior commissure, which join the inferior portions of the two temporal lobes and which have been followed in all the intervening plates from Figure 31 on. The diffuse fibers are the anterior forceps of the anterior commissure. These axons arise from neurons in the olfactory bulb, pass through the olfactory tract, diverge from it as the anterior forceps, cross in the decussation of the anterior commissure (305), and terminate in the contralateral olfactory bulb. Most of the fibers in an olfactory tract do not cross. They either diverge medially and terminate in the ipsilateral paraterminal gyrus (462) and subcallosal area (463), collectively the septal area, or they diverge laterally to end in the prepyriform area in the extreme rostral and basal part of the temporal lobe and in the amygdaloid nucleus (427, Fig. 35). The prepyriform area, which is not included in the figures, is the region concerned with the crude perception of odors. The function of the fibers which diverge medially into the septal area is obscure.

Dorsal to the anterior commissure the columns of the fornix (403) are sectioned just as they emerge from the hypothalamus to become continuous with the body of the fornix in Figure 38. The body of the fornix (401) forms the dorsal and rostral boundary of an interventricular foramen (306). The fornix appears to be suspended from the corpus callosum (402) by the septum pellucidum (405). In this specimen, the two septa pellucida are fused, thereby eliminating the fifth ventricle,

an inappropriate name for what is part of the subarachnoid space.

The anterior thalamic nucleus (326) is a prominent elevation immediately ventrolateral to an interventricular foramen (306). The tela choroidea of the third ventricle (311) extends through the foramen to become the tela choroidea of the lateral ventricle (408). Most of the cerebrospinal fluid is formed in the lateral ventricles. Normally there is free movement of fluid from each lateral ventricle (406) into the third ventricle (307, Fig. 39), then through the cerebral aqueduct into the fourth ventricle (205 and 105, Fig. 39). From the fourth ventricle the fluid enters the subarachnoid space through two lateral foramina (147, Fig. 13) and one medial foramen.

The figure shows the two anterior cerebral arteries (404) united by the short anterior communicating artery (unlabeled) which completes the circle of Willis rostrally. The middle cerebral artery (428) is labeled in the lateral fissure of Sylvius.

The anterior limb (423) of the internal capsule is obvious between the caudate nucleus (435) and the putamen (419). The approximate position of the genu of the internal capsule (422), which is never obvious in transverse sections, is indicated.

305—Anterior commissure
306—Interventricular foramen
311—Tela choroidea of the third ventricle
326—Anterior nucleus of the thalamus
329—Anterior ventral nucleus of the thalamus
402—Body of the corpus callosum
403—Column of the fornix
404—Anterior cerebral artery
405—Septum pellucidum
421—Globus pallidus
422—Genu of the internal capsule
423—Anterior limb of the internal capsule
428—Middle cerebral artery
435—Body of the caudate nucleus
446—Corona radiata
462—Paraterminal gyrus
463—Subcallosal area

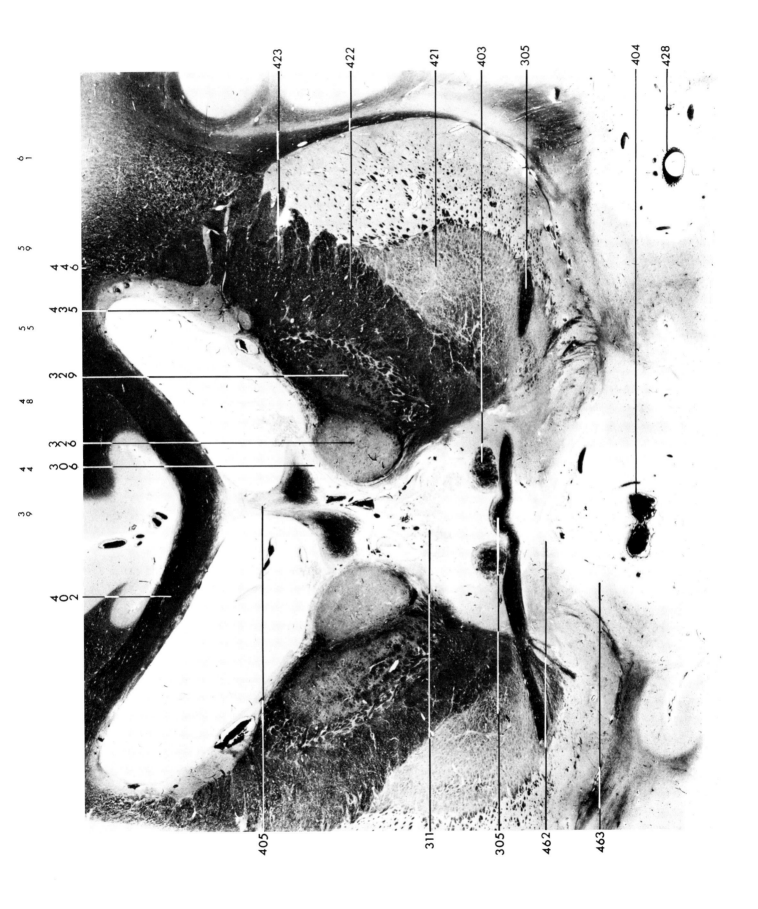

FIGURE 38. Junction of Body and Column of the Fornix

The final figure of the transverse series shows the continuity of the body (401) and column (403) of the fornix. Since the plane is wholly rostral of the thalamus, only the anterior limb of the internal capsule (423) is included. Frontopontine fibers and the reciprocal connections between the medial thalamic nucleus and the prefrontal cortex are the major constituents of the anterior limb. The head of the caudate nucleus (417) is labeled in two areas. If the section were a little farther rostral, it would be obvious that the head of the caudate is a single nuclear mass. The putamen (419) of the lentiform nucleus is likewise labeled twice to emphasize that ventral to the anterior commissure (305) it is continuous with the head of the caudate nucleus. The paraterminal gyrus (462) and subcallosal area (463), collectively the septal area, are obvious.

401—Body of the fornix
403—Column of the fornix
404—Anterior cerebral artery
405—Septum pellucidum
406—Body of the lateral ventricle
408—Tela choroidea of the lateral ventricle
417—Head of the caudate nucleus
419—Putamen
423—Anterior limb of the internal capsule
451—External capsule
456—Extreme capsule
457—Claustrum
462—Paraterminal gyrus
463—Subcallosal area

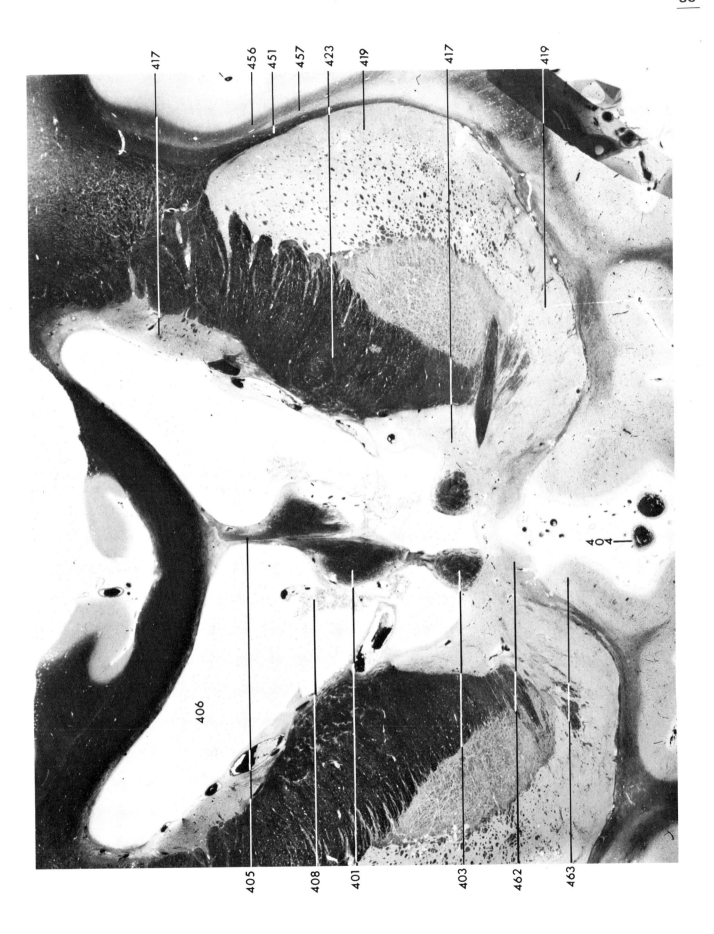

SAGITTAL

INTRODUCTION TO THE

Sagittal figures of the brain stem are more difficult to understand and interpret than transverse sections, but the effort is worthwhile for the development of a conception in three dimensions of the fiber tracts and nuclei.

The study of structures in sagittal and parasagittal sections after the transverse figures requires some reorientation of thinking. It is necessary first of all to have in mind how far any parasagittal section being studied is from the midsagittal plane, then to recollect how far from the midline any tract or nucleus was in a transverse section, and, finally, to think of the level of that transverse section in relation to the parasagittal section. A midsagittal section causes the least difficulty, because anyone who has studied transverse figures can name the sequence of structures in the midline at a transverse level of the medulla ob-

longata, pons, mesencephalon, or thalamus. It is less easy to recollect a similar sequence of structures, for example, 2 cm from the midline in a transverse section at the level of the facial colliculus, or at any other level of the brain.

To facilitate meeting these requirements, the planes of representative transverse figures (7 to 37) are shown on the parasagittal section that precedes Figure 1. In addition, at the top of each of these particular representative transverse sections (Figs. 7 to 37), the planes of the midsagittal (Fig. 39) and selected parasagittal (Figs. 44, 48, 55, etc.) sections are shown (*small numbers*). To illustrate their use, in Figure 10 a vertical line dropped from the small number 44 would traverse the structures visible in the medullary portion of sagittal Figure 44. Similarly, in Figure 20, a vertical line dropped from the small number 44

SAGITTAL FIGURES

would traverse the structures visible in Figure 44 at the level of the mesencephalon.

The parasagittal planes indicated in the transverse figures are not completely accurate because of differences in size and proportions between the two brains. For example, the sagittal brain lacked an intrathalamic adhesion, and the widths of the two third ventricles are not the same. These discrepancies between planes are greatest in the lateral parts of the diencephalon and telencephalon.

To the uninitiated it is sometimes disappointing to find that the great ascending and descending fiber tracts are not conspicuous in sagittal sections. This is because most fiber tracts do not run rostrocaudally in one plane but, instead, follow an oblique course, so that in a sagittal figure the fiber tract is cut obliquely rather than longi-

tudinally. A good example of this is the solitary fasciculus (18) in Figures 41 to 45. Almost the only tract which extends throughout the length of the brain stem in the same sagittal plane is the medial longitudinal fasciculus (8, Fig. 39). Although the medial lemniscus follows a straight caudal-rostral course in the medulla (10, Figs. 9 to 14), it is oblique in the rest of its course.

Cranial nerve nuclei also are disappointingly inconspicuous in sagittal sections. This must be accepted as a fact for which there is no ready explanation. As compensation, however, blood vessels are more conspicuous in sagittal than in transverse figures.

The cerebellum has been labeled minimally, because to have done more would not have been particularly helpful and would have made labeling of the medulla and pons less clear, owing to lack of space.

FIGURE 39.

A midsagittal section includes constituents of all five of the major subdivisions of the brain. Caudally, in the so called closed portion of the medulla, the ascending primary fibers of the gracile fasciculus (2) which terminate in the pale central gray matter. Ventral to these is the decussation of the pyramids (4), where descending corticospinal fibers course dorsally and caudally, cross to the opposite side, and descend throughout the entire length of the lateral corticospinal tract (37, Figs. 6 to 1). Caudal and ventral to the decussation is the anterior corticospinal tract (1). This is made up of motor fibers which do not cross in the pyramidal decussation but descend into the anterior funiculus in the upper part of the spinal cord (Fig. 6), where most of them do cross in the anterior white commissure. Rostral to the decussation of the pyramids, corticospinal fibers diverge laterally into the pyramids. Hence, in an absolutely precise midsagittal section the pyramids would not be seen as they are here.

In the "open" part of the medulla, the roof of the fourth ventricle (105) is in fact the posterior medullary velum and its tela choroidea (12). Between the fourth ventricle and the pyramids, three fiber tracts form a single mass of longitudinally oriented fibers. The most dorsal, the medial longitudinal fasciculus (8), extends from the mesencephalon through the pons and medulla into the cervical and upper thoracic spinal cord, where it is sometimes called the sulcomarginal tract. The medial longitudinal fasciculus is not sharply distinct from the tectospinal tract (9) in the medulla; in the midpons, however, the latter departs from the midsagittal plane and hence disappears from this figure, leaving the medial longitudinal fasciculus isolated in the rostral brain stem. Far more important than the tectospinal tract is the medial lemniscus (10), which occupies the triangular space between the pyramids and the tectospinal tract, with its apex directed caudally. Beyond the rostral end of the medulla, where the medial lemniscus is no longer confined by the inferior olive, the lemniscus shifts laterally and disappears from the midsagittal plane.

The numerous vertical white slashes in the medulla are branches of the anterior spinal artery, itself a branch of the vertebral artery; they supply the hypoglossal nucleus (6) and its fibers, the medial lemniscus, decussation of the pyramids, and pyramids. A lesion of the branches of the anterior spinal artery here can result in a crossed motor paralysis (see legend for Fig. 10) with sensory deficits, or a quadriplegia if the decussation of the pyramids (4) is involved.

The metencephalon includes the cerebellum and the basilar portions of the pons. The major fissures and divisions of the vermis in the cerebellum are identified here, but not in most of the following illustrations. The basilar pons is constituted in large measure of innumerable pale staining pontine nuclei (104) and pontocerebellar fibers (103) which arise in these pontine nuclei, run transversely, and cross into the contralateral basilar pons. There is little to identify in the tegmentum of the pons except for the medial longitudinal fasciculus and tectospinal tract; there are nuclei of the reticular formation which, however, cannot be identified specifically in these sections.

The basilar artery (102) is a midline vessel which arises through the fusion of the two vertebral arteries at the caudal end of the basilar pons and which divides dichotomously into two posterior cerebral arteries (407, Fig. 44) at the rostral end of the pons. Many unnamed midline branches traverse and supply the tegmental and basilar pons, as shown here.

Another major decussation is the decussation of the superior cerebellar peduncle (200) in the caudal end of the mesencephalic tegmentum, actually at the transverse level of the inferior colliculus (209, Fig. 41); however, because the colliculus is located parasagittally, it cannot be seen here in the tectum of the mesencephalon (204). The tectum is the roof of the cerebral aqueduct (205). The oculomotor complex of nuclei (201) occupies the tegmentum of the rostral mesencephalon, at the level of the superior colliculi (210, Fig. 41).

Numerous small posteromedial striate arteries (202) arise from the posterior cerebral arteries and pierce the posterior perforated substance to supply such structures as the oculomotor nuclei (201) and fibers, the mamillary nuclei (300), and the laterally situated crus cerebri (220, Fig. 46). Interruption of this blood supply occasions a crossed paralysis, involving the oculomotor nerve and corticospinal fibers in the crus cerebri (Weber's syndrome). Additional comment is in the legend for Figure 24.

Since almost the entire diencephalon is located lateral to the third ventricle (307) and its tela choroidea (311), little except decussating diencephalic fibers occurs in this figure. These include most importantly the optic chiasm (302) and the posterior (309), anterior (305), and habenular (310) commissures. The lamina terminalis (304), extending between the anterior commissure and the optic chiasm, is the rostral end of the prosencephalon in the midline. The pineal gland (308) is a part of the epithalamus, the mamillary body (300) is hypothalamus, and the transected infundibular stalk (301) of the hypophysis is a downgrowth of the hypothalamus.

Telencephalic derivatives are limited to two parts of the corpus callosum (400 and 402) and two parts of the fornix (401 and 403).

The communication between the fourth ventricle (105) and the cisterna magna (11) via the medial foramen is here artifactually enlarged. Communication between the lateral ventricles and the third ventricle (307) is via two interventricular foramina (306).

1—Anterior corticospinal tract
2—Gracile fasciculus
3—Gracile nucleus
4—Decussation of the pyramids
5—Dorsal longitudinal fasciculus
6—Hypoglossal nucleus
8—Medial longitudinal fasciculus
9—Tectospinal tract
10—Medial lemniscus
11—Cisterna magna
12—Tela choroidea of the fourth ventricle
100—Posterolateral fissure
101—Decussation of the trapezoid body
102—Basilar artery
103—Pontocerebellar fibers
104—Pontine nuclei
105—Fourth ventricle
106—Nodulus
107—Uvula
108—Tonsil
109—Pyramis
110—Tuber
111—Folium
112—Declive
113—Primary fissure
114—Culmen
115—Central lobule
116—Lingula
200—Decussation of the superior cerebellar peduncles
201—Oculomotor nucleus
202—Posteromedial striate arteries
203—Decussation of the trochlear nerve
204—Tectum
205—Cerebral aqueduct
300—Mamillary nucleus
301—Infundibular stalk
302—Optic chiasm
303—Optic recess
304—Lamina terminalis
305—Anterior commissure
306—Interventricular foramen
307—Third ventricle
308—Pineal body
309—Posterior commissure
310—Habenular commissure
311—Tela choroidea of the third ventricle
400—Splenium of the corpus callosum
401—Body of the fornix
402—Body of the corpus callosum
403—Column of the fornix
404—Anterior cerebral artery

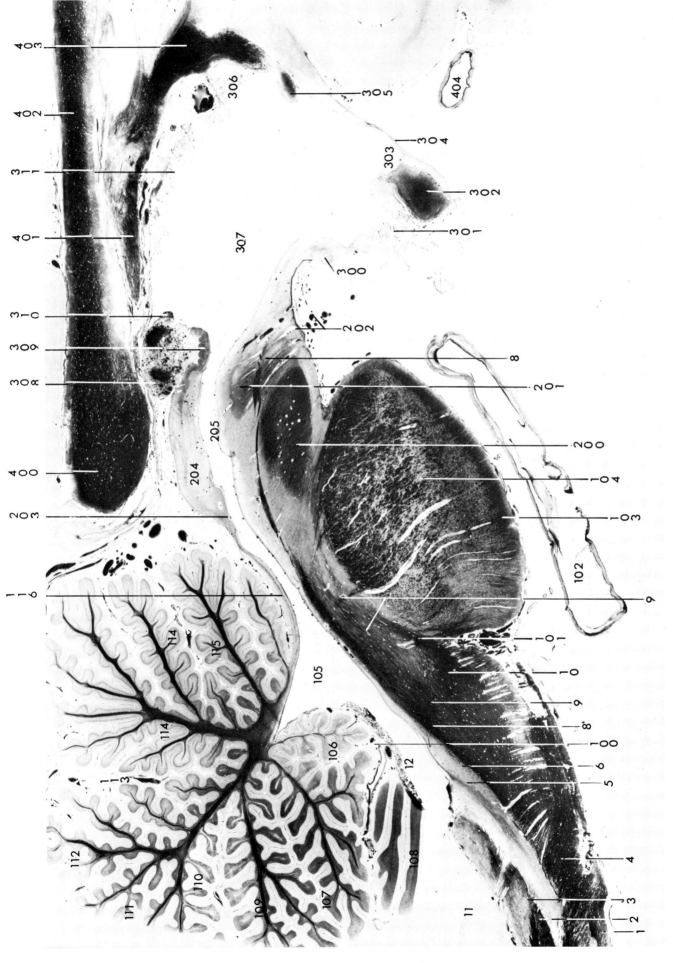

FIGURE 40.

1—Anterior corticospinal tract
2—Gracile fasciculus
3—Gracile nucleus
4—Decussation of the pyramids
5—Dorsal longitudinal fasciculus
6—Hypoglossal nucleus
8—Medial longitudinal fasciculus
9—Tectospinal tract
10—Medial lemniscus
11—Cisterna magna
12—Tela choroidea of the fourth ventricle
13—Internal arcuate fibers
14—Pyramid
102—Basilar artery
103—Pontocerebellar fibers
104—Pontine nuclei
105—Fourth ventricle
113—Primary fissure
117—Trapezoid body
118—Corticospinal fibers
119—Anterior medullary velum
200—Decussation of the superior cerebellar peduncles
201—Oculomotor nucleus
203—Decussation of the trochlear nerve
204—Tectum
205—Cerebral aqueduct
206—Interpeduncular fossa
300—Mamillary nucleus
301—Infundibular stalk
304—Lamina terminalis
306—Interventricular foramen
309—Posterior commissure
310—Habenular commissure
311—Tela choroidea of the third ventricle
312—Median eminence
402—Body of the corpus callosum
403—Column of the fornix
405—Septum pellucidum

The origin of the medial lemniscus (10) can be visualized in Figure 40. Axons of neurons located in the gracile nucleus (3) sweep laterally in a semicircular path around the central gray matter, where they are called internal arcuate fibers (13) since they cross the midline, and accumulate as the medial lemniscus, dorsal to the contralateral pyramid (14). Figures 8 and 9 show internal arcuate fibers in a transverse section.

The medial lemniscus is at first small, but as more and more fibers enter it the lemniscus assumes the shape of a wedge in a sagittal section. The first fibers entering the lemniscus receive impulses initiated in the most inferior parts of the lower extremity. Subsequent internal arcuate fibers, at first from the gracile nucleus and then from the cuneate nucleus, accumulate dorsal to those already in the medial lemniscus. Hence, the localization of fibers is as if one side of a headless homunculus were standing upon a pyramid (14); the right hemihomunculus stands upon the left pyramid and *vice versa*.

At the junction of the medulla and pons the medial lemniscus rounds up and then flattens into a broad band (in the transverse plane) in the ventral pontine tegmentum. This is obvious in transverse sections (Figs. 14 to 18), but is less easily visualized in this and the previous sagittal section. As this tape-like medial lemniscus ascends through the tegmentum of the pons and mesencephalon it slowly shifts laterally. Hence, in this and the following parasagittal sections, the medial lemniscus (10) in the pons is cut obliquely and occupies an ever more rostral position in the ventral tegmentum immediately adjacent to the basilar pons. Its position in the mesencephalon and its ultimate termination in the posterolateral ventral thalamic nucleus will be considered in later legends.

The entire rostral-caudal extent of the pyramid is now included in this section. The most medial of the corticospinal fibers (118) in the basilar pons are just appearing, and their continuity with pyramidal fibers will be established in the following figures.

The mesencephalon and thalamus display no notable changes except 'for a larger segment of the mamillary body (300), one of the large hypothalamic nuclei. The fornix is a major source of afferent fibers to the mamillary nucleus. It includes the body of the fornix (401), which is dorsal to the tela choroidea (311) of the third ventricle (307) and which curves ventrally to form the anterior edge of the interventricular foramen, where it becomes the column of the fornix (403, Fig. 45). The column of the fornix passes caudal to the anterior commissure (305, Fig. 45), courses through the hypothalamus (403, Fig. 46, and terminates in the mamillary body (300). The body of the fornix (401) hangs beneath the corpus callosum (402) as if suspended by the membranous septum pellucidum (405), which forms the medial wall of the rostral part of the lateral ventricle. Caudally, the fornix passes out of the section as it curves laterally, then caudally and inferiorly, to its origin in the hippocampus. This origin is seen in the most lateral of the sagittal sections (Fig. 63); its course can be followed in the intervening sections. Thus, the origin of the fornix is in the hippocampus, while its major terminations are the mamillary nucleus, septal area, and preoptic hypothalamus.

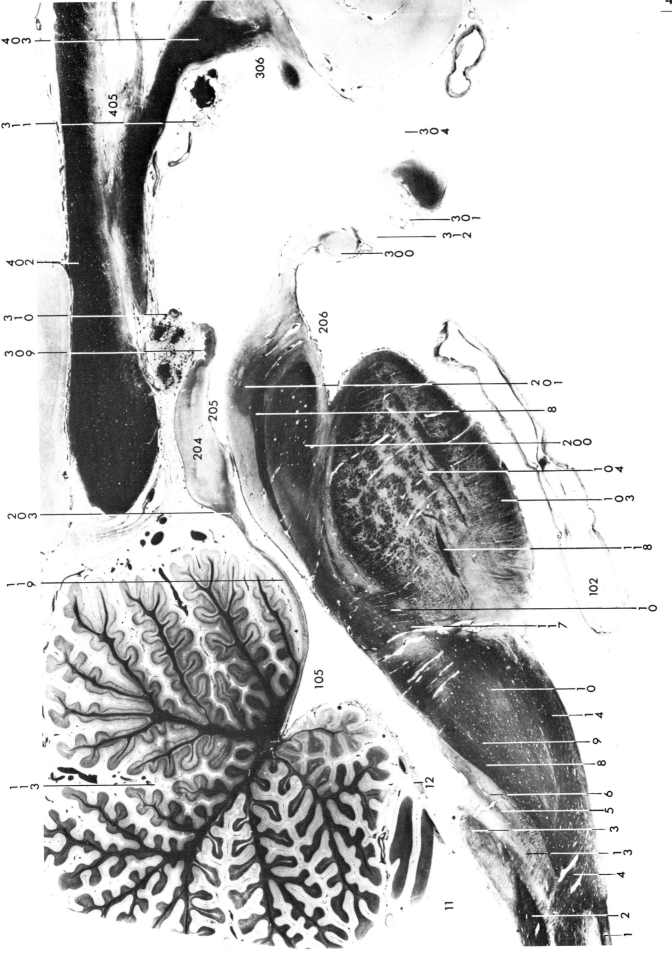

403
405
306
31
304
301
312
300
42
310
309
206
204
205
201
8
200
104
103
18
102
23
10
19
7
105
13
12
11
10
14
9
8
6
5
3
13
4
2
1

FIGURE 41.

Most of the major changes are confined to the medulla oblongata. The cuneate nucleus (21) occupies a seemingly aberrant position ventral and caudal of the gracile fasciculus (2) and nucleus (3), but reference to Figure 9 will clarify how both nuclei can be included in a single sagittal section. Oblique segments of the internal arcuate fibers (13), which arise now from both these nuclei, can be traced ventrally toward the medial lemniscus (10). The most medial of the fibers of the medial longitudinal fasciculus (8) and tectospinal tract (9) lie ventral to the cuneate nucleus. This figure shows how fibers which seem to be quite dorsal in the medulla (Fig. 9) and pons come to occupy the anterior funiculus in the spinal cord (Figs. 5 and 6).

In addition to the hypoglossal nucleus (6), the figure includes the dorsal nucleus of the vagus nerve (17) and the solitary nucleus and tract (18). Here, in the closed portion of the medulla, the dorsal vagal nucleus, which gives origin to the vagal preganglionic fibers, occupies a position dorsal to the somatic motor hypoglossal nucleus, just as in the spinal cord the visceral motor column lies dorsal to the somatic motor (N and J, Fig. 4). In the open part of the medulla a medial-lateral relationship obtains, but this is obvious only in transverse sections.

The solitary tract and nucleus (18) are sectioned obliquely for reasons explained in the introduction to the sagittal figures. In the following figures they occupy progressively more rostral postions. The caudal end of the tract contains all the primary general visceral afferent fibers of cranial nerves VII, IX, and X (and only these) while the rostral end of the tract contains special visceral afferent fibers of taste in addition to the descending general visceral fibers. Secondary fibers from the solitary nucleus which must exist to mediate reflex and sensory connections are not well understood. Many believe the sensory fibers

(largely those mediating taste) ascend as a component of the medial lemniscus.

The pyramids (14) end abruptly at the caudal end of the medulla as the corticospinal fibers pass medially out of the section toward their decussation, as already seen in previous figures. In the basilar pons there are many longitudinally oriented corticospinal fibers (118), and some can be followed into the pyramids.

In the mesencephalon, the plane of the figure is now lateral to the cerebral aqueduct but still includes a considerable segment of the medial longitudinal fasciculus (8) where it cradles the oculomotor nucleus (201). Most of the ascending fibers of the medial longitudinal fasciculus in the mesencephalon terminate in the trochlear (208, Fig. 42) or oculomotor (201) nuclei. Ventral to the latter, the most medial of the oculomotor fibers (207) slant rostrally toward the interpeduncular fossa (206). The fossa is the large space between the basilar pons and the mamillary nucleus (300).

The decussation of the superior cerebellar peduncle (211) lies ventral to the inferior colliculus (209), but here it is not distinct from the pedundular fibers which course rostrally beyond the decussation.

In the hypothalamus, the origin of the mamillothalamic fasciculus (313) is a small group of fibers on the dorsal and rostral aspect of the mamillary nucleus (300). Via this fasciculus impulses, coming in part from the hippocampus over fibers of the fornix (401 and 403), are projected to the anterior thalamic nucleus (326, Fig. 46); this will become apparent in the following figures.

The median eminence (312) contains axonal endings of neurons which synthesize the hormones that facilitate or inhibit the release of the trophic hormones of the adenohypophysis. The primary plexus of vessels of the hypophyseal portal system covers the surface of the median eminence. These vessels convey the hypothalamic hormones directly to the adeno-hypophysis.

1—Anterior corticospinal tract
2—Gracile fasciculus
3—Gracile nucleus
6—Hypoglossal nucleus
8—Medial longitudinal fasciculus
9—Tectospinal tract
10—Medial lemniscus
12—Tela choroidea of the fourth ventricle
13—Internal arcuate fibers
14—Pyramid
15—Medial accessory olivary nucleus
16—Inferior olivary nucleus
17—Dorsal nucleus of the vagus nerve
18—Nucleus and tractus solitarius
21—Cuneate nucleus
105—Fourth ventricle
117—Trapezoid body
118—Corticospinal fibers
119—Anterior medullary velum
201—Oculomotor nuclei
207—Oculomotor fibers
209—Inferior colliculus
210—Superior colliculus
211—Superior cerebellar peduncle
212—Trochlear fibers
302—Optic chiasm
303—Optic recess
304—Lamina terminalis
305—Anterior commissure
307—Third ventricle
308—Pineal body
310—Habenular commissure
311—Tela choroidea of the third ventricle
312—Median eminence
313—Mamillothalamic fasciculus
400—Splenium of the corpus callosum
401—Body of the fornix
403—Column of the fornix
404—Anterior cerebral artery

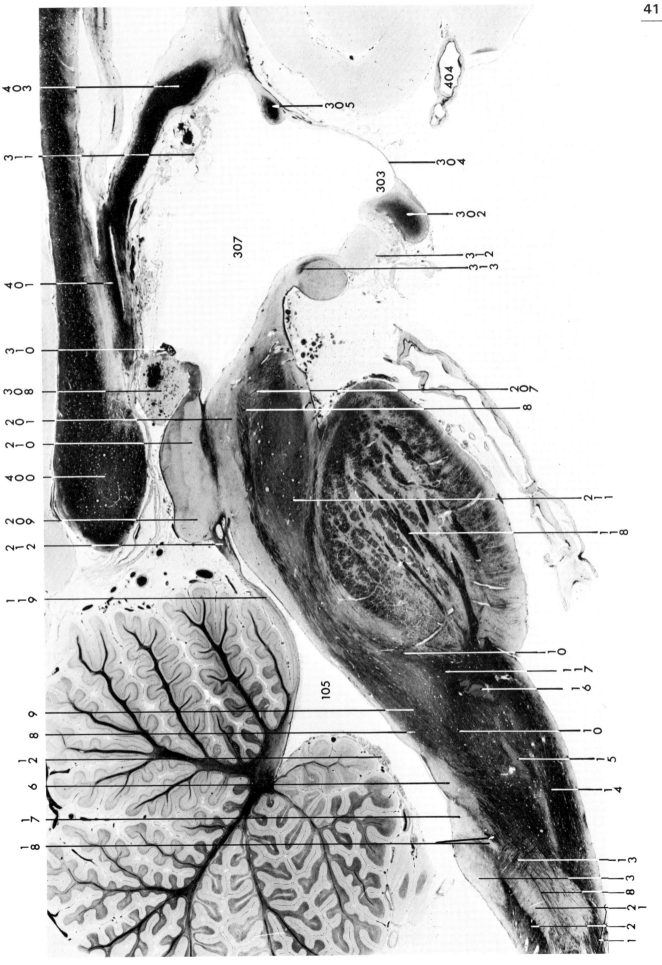

FIGURE 42.

There are few new developments in the medulla. In addition to the cuneate nucleus (21), the section includes the ascending primary fibers of the fasciculus cuneatus (20), which convey impulses initiated in tactile receptors and in receptors in muscles, tendons, and joints of the upper part of the body on the ipsilateral side to the cuneate nucleus. More rostrally in the medulla, several groups of fibers of the hypoglossal nerve (22) are passing ventrally at right angles to the medial longitudinal fasciculus (8) and tectospinal tract (9), but are seen only for a short distance because they course laterally, and hence leave the plane of this section to emerge between the pyramid and the inferior olive. In the area of the trapezoid body (117) the section is quite dark where these transverse auditory fibers interdigitate with the longitudinally coursing fibers of the medial lemniscus (10). Far lateral to this section, where the trapezoid fibers turn and assume a longitudinal course, they become known as the lateral lemniscus (136 in the ventral pontine tegmentum, Fig. 47), and as such can be followed as they course dorsolaterally around the superior cerebellar peduncle (Figs. 47 to 51) and then curve dorsomedially (136 in the dorsal pontine tegmentum, Figs. 51 to 46) to their major termination in the inferior colliculus (209, Fig. 46).

The most medial of the deep nuclei in the white matter of the cerebellum is the fastigial nucleus (120). It receives intracerebellar fibers from the cortex of the vermis, and primary vestibular fibers from outside the cerebellum via the juxtarestiform body. The juxtarestiform body, which also contains efferent fibers arising in the fastigial nucleus, is a more lateral structure and will be identified in Figures 48 and 49. Fastigial fibers terminate in the vestibular and reticular nuclei.

The basilar pons here consists of the widely scattered, lightly staining pontine nuclei (104) and two groups of fibers. The longitudinally oriented fibers are, collectively, the corticospinal, corticobulbar, and corticopontine fibers. Only on the basis of their closeness to the pyramids is it possible to designate some as corticospinal (118). Corticopontine fibers convey impulses from the cerebral cortex to the pontine nuclei (104) where they synapse. Axons issue from the pontine nuclei to form the pontocerebellar fibers (103), which are the transected bundles of fibers lying dorsal and ventral to the central, longitudinal fibers in the basilar pons. These pontocerebellar fibers gradually converge laterally into a compact bundle, the middle cerebellar peduncle, which sweeps dorsally into the cerebellum (142, Figs. 50 to 54).

In the mesencephalon, the trochlear nucleus (208) indents the medial longitudinal fasciculus (8) at the transverse level of the inferior colliculus (209). Since the trochlear fibers decussate in the anterior medullary velum immediately caudal to the inferior colliculus (203, Fig. 39), it is obvious that trochlear fibers must slant caudally as they follow a semicircular path around the central gray matter.

In the interpeduncular fossa (206), which is the space bounded laterally by the cerebral peduncles, there are numerous unlabeled branches of the posteromedial striate arteries, some seen entering the brain in the region called the posterior perforated substance. This section now includes not only the floor of the hypothalamus but also part of the lateral walls which slope into it. The tela choroidea of the third ventricle (311) is labeled close to where it extends through the interventricular foramen (306) to become the tela choroidea of the lateral ventricles (408, Fig. 45).

The basilar artery (102) is sectioned along its lateral edge and hence appears to be interrupted. At the rostral end of the artery is the slender stump (unlabeled) of what is probably a posterior communicating artery.

1—Anterior corticospinal tract
2—Gracile fasciculus
3—Gracile nucleus
6—Hypoglossal nucleus
8—Medial longitudinal fasciculus
9—Tectospinal tract
10—Medial lemniscus
11—Cisterna magna
13—Internal arcuate fibers
15—Medial accessory olivary nucleus
16—Inferior olivary nucleus
17—Dorsal nucleus of the vagus nerve
18—Nucleus and tractus solitarius
20—Cuneate fasciculus
21—Cuneate nucleus
22—Hypoglossal fibers
102—Basilar artery
103—Pontocerebellar fibers
104—Pontine nuclei
117—Trapezoid body
118—Corticospinal fibers
119—Anterior medullary velum
120—Fastigial nucleus
201—Oculomotor nucleus
206—Interpeduncular fossa
207—Oculomotor fibers
208—Trochlear nucleus
209—Inferior colliculus
211—Superior cerebellar peduncle
300—Mamillary nucleus
304—Lamina terminalis
306—Interventricular foramen
309—Posterior commissure
310—Habenular commissure
311—Tela choroidea of the third ventricle
312—Median eminence
400—Splenium of the corpus callosum
402—Body of the corpus callosum
406—Body of the lateral ventricle

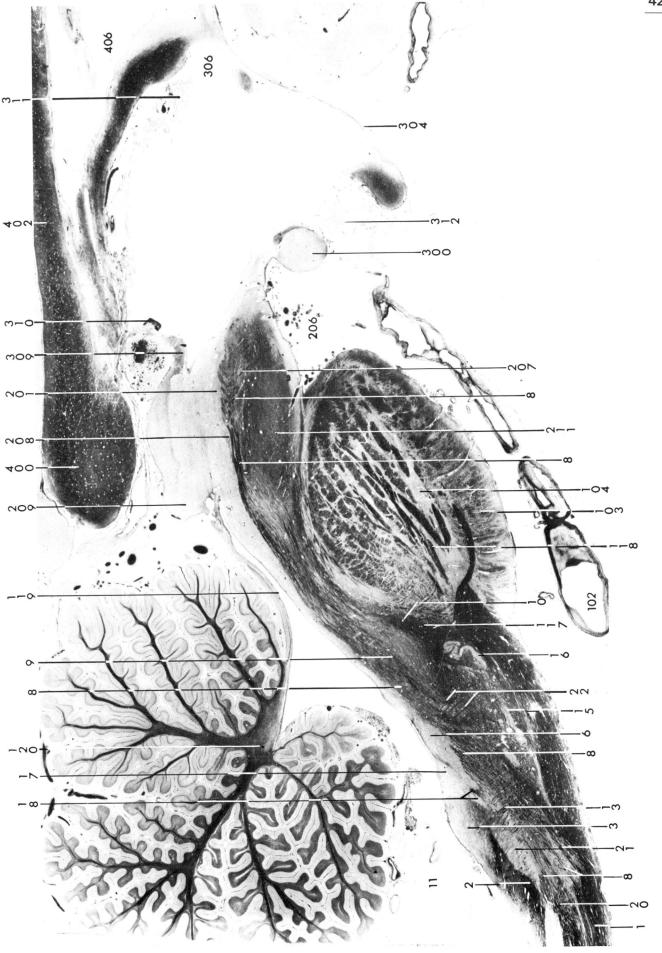

FIGURE 43.

In the medulla, the gracile (3) and hypoglossal (6) nuclei are sectioned through their lateral sides and hence appear diminished in size. The hypoglossal nucleus would scarcely be distinguishable from the other gray matter in the floor of the fourth ventricle (105) except for the myelinated fibers of the dorsal longitudinal fasciculus (5) which cover it dorsally.

A large portion of the inferior olive (16) is visible. Seemingly in its ventral part are the fibers of the hypoglossal nerve (22). Because these fibers curve laterally to become superficial between the pyramid (14) and the inferior olive, they are cut obliquely in this sagittal section. Reference to transverse Figure 12, where hypoglossal fibers are visible, just lateral of the medial lemniscus, makes these relations clear. Fibers of the abducens nerve (146) are prominent in the tegmentum in the caudal part of the pons. They emerge from the medial side of the abducens nucleus, which therefore is visible only in the next figure. In this section, abducens fibers course ventrally and caudally into the dark mass of fibers at the rostral end of the inferior olive, where fibers of the medial lemniscus and the trapezoid body interdigitate. The abducens nerve becomes superficial at the caudal border of the pons.

The fibers running rostrocaudally in the basilar pons include corticopontine, corticobulbar, and corticospinal fibers. They are indistinguishably mingled except for corticospinal fibers (118), which alone enter the pyramid (14). The anterior medullary velum (119), forming in part the roof of the fourth ventricle (105), is still thin and devoid of fibers, in marked contrast to the same velum in Figure 44. There are no significant changes in the mesencephalon.

In the diencephalon the pineal gland (308) appears smaller as the plane of section passes through its lateral portion. Only the most lateral edge of it appears in the next section. The dorsal part of the thalamus proper is now included in the section for the first time. Although labeled the medial nucleus (317), the *leader* may actually be terminating in the old midline nuclei of the thalamus. Dorsal to the medial nucleus are the longitudinally oriented fibers of the stria medullaris of the thalamus (316). These fibers, which have several origins, synapse in the habenular nuclei (315, Fig. 45). The stria medullaris follow a slightly semicircular course in the horizontal plane so that the middle part appears first in a sagittal series while the rostral and caudal ends of the stria are included in the following sections. Ventrally, the optic nerve (314) makes its initial appearance in the sagittal figures.

The lateral ventricle (406) is now unencumbered by any portion of the septum pellucidum. The illustration includes both the body and the anterior horn of the lateral ventricle. The anterior horn is that portion which lies rostral to the interventricular foramen (306).

3—Gracile nucleus
5—Dorsal longitudinal fasciculus
6—Hypoglossal nucleus
8—Medial longitudinal fasciculus
10—Medial lemniscus
13—Internal arcuate fibers
14—Pyramid
16—Inferior olivary nucleus
18—Nucleus and tractus solitarius
22—Hypoglossal fibers
102—Basilar artery
105—Fourth ventricle
113—Primary fissure
118—Corticospinal fibers
119—Anterior medullary velum
120—Fastigial nucleus
146—Abducens fibers
206—Interpeduncular fossa
210—Superior colliculus
211—Superior cerebellar peduncle
302—Optic chiasm
303—Optic recess
304—Lamina terminalis
305—Anterior commissure
307—Third ventricle
308—Pineal body
313—Mamillothalamic fasciculus
314—Optic nerve
316—Stria medullaris of the thalamus
317—Medial (dorsal medial) nucleus of the thalamus
401—Body of the fornix
404—Anterior cerebral artery
406—Body of the lateral ventricle

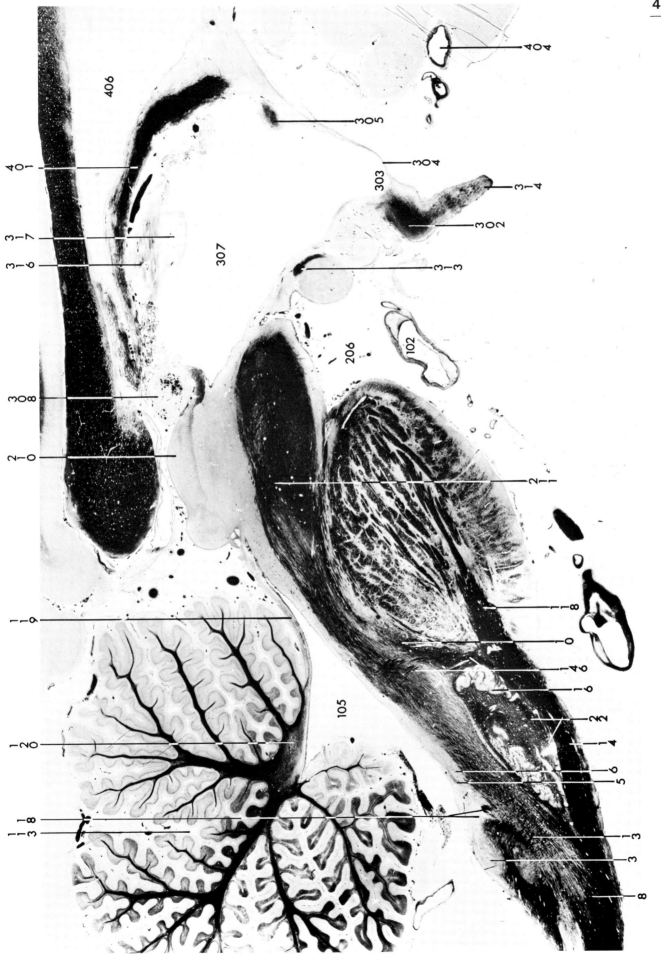

FIGURE 44.

Figure 44 is the first sagittal section to include the spinal trigeminal nucleus (19) and tract (25). Reference to these two elongated structures in the transverse series of the medulla (Figs. 7 to 14) shows that the nucleus is always medial to the tract and that as the medulla increases in size they retain a superficial position in the brain stem. Hence, in sagittal sections such as this, the nucleus and tract are sectioned obliquely, just as are the nucleus and tractus solitarius (18). This is the major new development, since the connections and function of the arcuate nucleus (7) are not understood; arcuate fibers extend into the cerebellum. The reticular formation (34) is the extensive area of longitudinally oriented myelinated fibers interspersed with diffuse nuclei dorsal to the inferior olive, here and in Figures 43 and 45. The axon of a reticular neuron characteristically divides into a long ascending and a long descending branch.

The abducens nucleus (121), the source of motor fibers to the lateral rectus muscle of the eye, is also the most caudal landmark in the pontine tegmentum, thereby establishing the transition from myelencephalon to metencephalon dorsally, just as the pons does ventrally. The origin and course of the branchiomeric motor fibers of the facial nerve have been described in the legend to Figure 16. In this figure the fibers of the internal genu of the facial nerve (122) are transected as they curve laterally around the rostral end of the abducens nucleus.

The medial lemniscus (10) is sectioned obliquely in the tegmentum of the pons. The gradual rostral shift in the position of each segment of the fillet as it extends to the thalamus is more readily perceived by comparing Figures 41 and 46 with this figure. In the basilar pons the plane of the section passes through the very middle of the corticospinal fibers (118). The more dorsal, longitudinally sectioned fibers are corticopontine tracts (124) that synapse in the pontine nuclei (104), which in turn project pontocerebellar fibers (103) to the contralateral cerebellum via the middle cerebellar peduncle (142, Figs. 50 to 56).

The medial edge of the superior cerebellar peduncle is included here in the anterior medullary velum, which was devoid of fibers in more medial figures. This fiber tract has lateral origins in globose (126, Fig. 45). emboliform (130, Fig. 46), and dentate (137, Fig. 50) nuclei, and Figure 14. Hence the peduncle necessarily courses medially as well as rostrally to its decussation (200, Fig. 39). Rostral of the decussation, the peduncle diverges laterally (211 in the mesencephalon) and synapses in the red nucleus (214), intermediate ventral, anterior ventral, and some intralaminar nuclei (337, 329, Fig. 55). The ventral nuclei are an intermediate synapse in the main pathway between the cerebellum and the frontal lobes of the cerebral cortex. The red nucleus projects fibers to the inferior olivary (16) and reticular nuclei (34) in the brain-stem via the central tegmental tract (123, Fig. 45) and to the spinal cord. Rubrothalamic fibers are less well established.

The habenular nucleus (315) lies caudally in the epithalamus, just rostral to the pineal body (308). Most of the afferent fibers to the habenula reach it via the stria medullaris of the thalamus (316), which is here labeled in two places where it passes in and out of the section as it curves around the medial nucleus (317). Fibers of the stria originate in the septal area, anterior thalamic nucleus, and hippocampus. Some cross in the habenular commissure (310, Figs. 39 to 42). Efferent habenular fibers form the fasciculus retroflexus (318, Figs. 27, 28, and 45 to 48) that synapses in the interpeduncular nucleus (213) and in tegmental nuclei in the mesencephalon.

Although the basilar artery is no longer included in the figure, the vertebral artery (23), which fuses with its opposite number to form the basilar artery, is included, along with the terminal branch of the basilar artery, the posterior cerebral artery (407) and the paraterminal branch, the superior cerebellar artery (125). These last two vessels take a semicircular course around the brain stem parallel to each other (Figs. 45 to 47), then diverge to supply the cerebellum and cerebrum as indicated by their names. They also have branches that are distributed to the colliculi and the thalamus. One of a number of vessels, collectively called anteromedial striate vessels (409), is labeled close to its origin from the anterior cerebral artery (404). They supply the rostral portions of the corpus striatum and the internal capsule.

7—Arcuate nucleus
10—Medial lemniscus
11—Cisterna magna
12—Tela choroidea of the fourth ventricle
13—Internal arcuate fibers
17—Dorsal nucleus of the vagus nerve
18—Nucleus and tractus solitarius
19—Spinal trigeminal nucleus
20—Cuneate fasciculus
21—Cuneate nucleus
23—Vertebral artery
25—Spinal tract of the trigeminal nerve
34—Reticular formation
103—Pontocerebellar fibers
104—Pontine nuclei
117—Trapezoid body
118—Corticospinal fibers
120—Fastigial nucleus
121—Abducens nucleus
122—Genu of the facial nerve
123—Central tegmental tract
124—Corticopontine fibers
125—Superior cerebellar artery
207—Oculomotor fibers
209—Inferior colliculus
211—Superior cerebellar peduncle
212—Trochlear fibers
213—Interpeduncular nucleus
214—Red nucleus
300—Mamillary nucleus
302—Optic chiasm
303—Optic recess
306—Interventricular foramen
309—Posterior commissure
315—Habenula
316—Stria medullaris of the thalamus
317—Medial (dorsal medial) nucleus of the thalamus
401—Body of the fornix
402—Body of the corpus callosum
403—Column of the fornix
407—Posterior cerebral artery
408—Tela choroidea of the lateral ventricle
409—Anteromedial striate artery

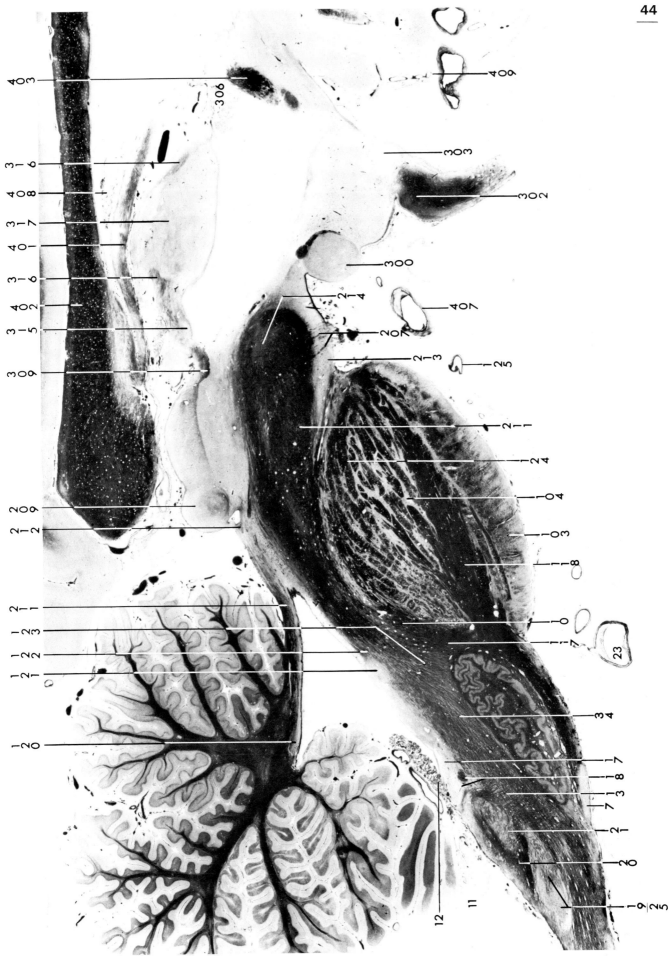

FIGURE 45.

The more slender caudal part of the medulla is no longer in the figure, and an oblique section of the spinal trigeminal nucleus (19) is the terminal structure. Only a little of the pyramid (14) and the cuneate nucleus (21) are still included, but internal arcuate fibers (13) are numerous. Two nuclei of the vestibular complex, the inferior (127) and medial (128), while lying dorsolateral to the solitary nucleus and tract (18), have been given pontine numbers since they secondarily invade the medulla. The nucleus ambiguus, which is too slender to be visible in this Weigert section, occupies a position in the reticular formation dorsal to the inferior olive. The nucleus ambiguus is about coextensive in length with the inferior olive rostrally, but extends beyond it into the caudal medulla.

The large central tegmental tract (123) is a dark longitudinal mass of fibers which follows the curvature of the basilar pons, encompasses the rostral pole of the inferior olivary nucleus (16), and spreads out to form a capsule over its dorsal surface before synapsing therein. The tract can be readily confused with the trapezoid fibers and the medial lemniscus in more medial sections, such as Figure 42. However, here the trapezoid fibers (117) are ventral to the central tegmental tract, while the medial lemniscus (10) is a slender semicircular band of obliquely sectioned fibers which has shifted to a more rostral position in the most ventral part of the pontine tegmentum.

A large segment of the superior cerebellar peduncle (211) is included in the anterior medullary velum, and a few fibers can be followed into the tegmentum ventral to the inferior colliculus (209). The peduncle extends rostrally on the lateral side of the central tegmental tract, and hence can be followed rostrally only in the following figures, but its relation to the central tegmental tract is per-

ceived better here and in Figure 19 of the transverse series.

Globose nuclei (126) are small, light areas in the cerebellar white matter. They contribute axons to the superior cerebellar peduncle. Ventral to the superior cerebellar peduncle are the processes of primary fibers which constitute the mesencephalic tract (129) of the trigeminal nerve. The accompanying mesencephalic nucleus is a major exception to the rule that the cell bodies of peripheral nerves are located in ganglia outside the central nervous system. The peripheral processes of the mesencephalic nucleus arise in receptors in the muscles of mastication and in the teeth. The tract can be followed in favorable material rostrally to the level of the superior colliculus, and it has been suggested that the mesencephalic tract may also contain the central processes of the perikarya which are scattered along the trochlear and oculomotor nerves and whose peripheral processes arise in receptors in the extrinsic ocular muscles. These receptors and fibers are of importance in the precise reflex adjustment of the two eyes.

Reference to Figure 23 will clarify how the periaqueductal gray matter (215) at the level of the superior colliculus can appear as a large nucleus in a sagittal section. Ventrally the medial corticobulbar fibers (216), the most medial of the fibers constituting the crus cerebri, are barely included in the section. Oculomotor fibers now converge, course through the red nucleus (214), and leave the brain stem as the oculomotor nerve (217).

The pretectal area (218), which is a center for optic reflexes mediated by smooth muscle, lies just beyond the rostral slope of the superior colliculus (210). This colliculus is a center mediating the reflex turning of the eyes, which is thus effected by skeletal muscles. Dorsal to the pretectal area is the ha-

benula (315), which receives fibers of the stria medullaris of the thalamus. The fasciculus retroflexus (318), which arises at least in part in the habenula and extends to the interpeduncular nucleus (213, Fig. 44), is sectioned close to its origin.

In the ventral part of the diencephalon, the plane of section now passes through the medial hypothalamic area. The medial area is roughly separated from the lateral hypothalamic area by the column of the fornix (403, Fig. 46), which plunges between them to terminate in the mamillary body (300). Figure 33 of the transverse series shows both medial and lateral hypothalamic areas in relation to the column of the fornix. Figure 48 shows the lateral hypothalamic area. The approximate positions of major nuclear masses (319 to 323) of the medial hypothalamic area are indicated in the present sagittal section.

10—Medial lemniscus
12—Tela choroidea of the fourth ventricle
13—Internal arcuate fibers
14—Pyramid
16—Inferior olivary nucleus
18—Nucleus and tractus solitarius
19—Spinal trigeminal nucleus
20—Cuneate fasciculus
21—Cuneate nucleus
105—Fourth ventricle
117—Trapezoid body
118—Corticospinal fibers
123—Central tegmental tract
125—Superior cerebellar artery
126—Globose nucleus
127—Inferior vestibular nucleus
128—Medial vestibular nucleus
129—Mesencephalic nucleus and tract of the trigeminal nerve
210—Superior colliculus
211—Superior cerebellar peduncle
212—Trochlear fibers
215—Periaqueductal gray matter
216—Medial corticobulbar fibers
217—Oculomotor nerve
218—Pretectal area
305—Anterior commissure
306—Interventricular foramen
307—Third ventricle
313—Mamillothalamic fasciculus
314—Optic nerve
315—Habenula
316—Stria medullaris of the thalamus
317—Medial (dorsal medial) nucleus of the thalamus
318—Fasciculus retroflexus
319—Posterior nucleus of the hypothalamus
320—Dorsomedial nucleus of the hypothalamus
321—Ventromedial nucleus of the hypothalamus
322—Supraoptic nucleus of the hypothalamus
323—Preoptic nucleus of the hypothalamus
324—Pulvinar
400—Splenium of the corpus callosum
401—Body of the fornix
403—Column of the fornix
404—Anterior cerebral artery
406—Body of the lateral ventricle
407—Posterior cerebral artery
408—Tela choroidea of the lateral ventricle
410—Crus of the fornix

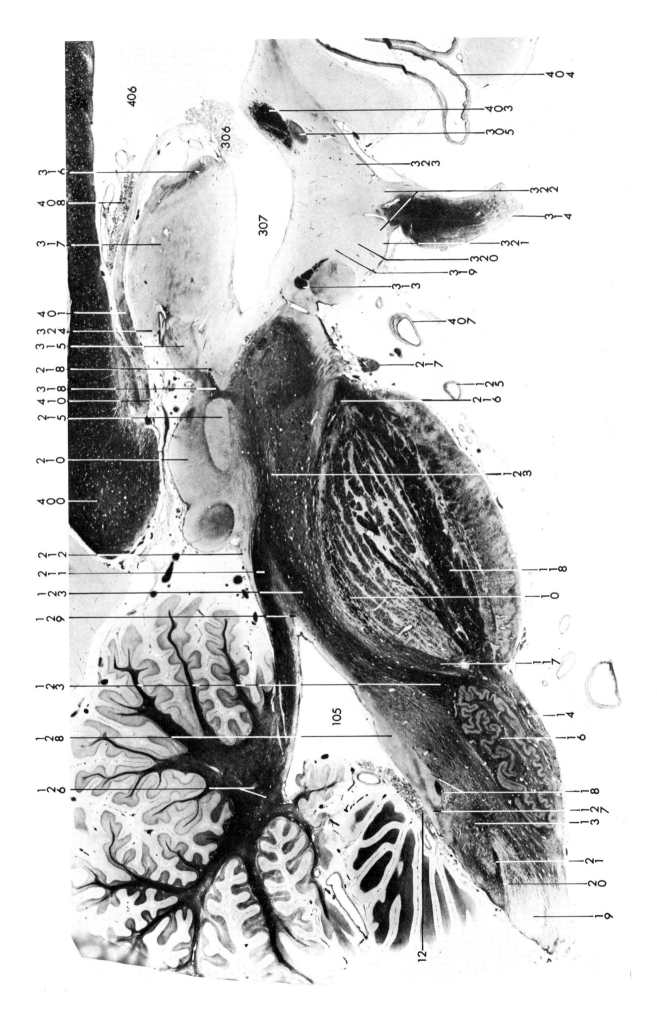

FIGURE 46.

The medulla now appears markedly truncated, but what remains includes the major tracts which ascend at the periphery of the medulla. Immediately ventral to the cuneate fasciculus (20) and its nucleus (21) is the spinal tract of the trigeminal nerve (25). The intermingled anterior spinocerebellar and spinothalamic tracts are among the longitudinally oriented fibers dorsal to the inferior olive (16).

Many components of the vestibular complex are present. The descending branches of primary fibers of the vestibular nerve (26) are coarse fibers in the dorsal region of the medulla. These fibers descend within the inferior vestibular nucleus and give it a speckled appearance in transverse sections (127, Fig. 13). Since these descending fibers synapse in the medial (128) and inferior vestibular nuclei, the number of myelinated fibers progressively diminishes caudally, and the terminal portion of the inferior nucleus becomes pale; it is this part of the nucleus which is labeled here (127). Immediately rostral to the descending vestibular fibers is the lateral vestibular nucleus (143). Lateral and superior (135) vestibular nuclei receive ascending primary vestibular fibers.

The motor nucleus of the facial nerve (131) is a prominent light area in the pontine tegmentum caudal to the trapezoid body (117), while rostral to it is the elongated and inconspicuous superior olive (132).

Auditory fibers, which course nearly transversely in the trapezoid body (117, Fig. 17), turn rostrally, approximately in the plane of the present figure, and follow a nearly longitudinally oriented course in the pons and mesencephalon; they are now designated the lateral lemniscus (136, Fig. 47). Spinothalamic fibers (133) mediating pain and temperature intermingle with or are adjacent to the auditory fibers of the lateral lemniscus. Most of the auditory fibers terminate in the

inferior colliculus (209). To reach this nucleus the lateral lemniscus swings laterally around the superior cerebellar peduncle (211) as it plunges into the tegmentum of the mesencephalon. Then the lateral lemniscus curves medially to terminate in the inferior colliculus; it is these medially directed lemniscal fibers (136) which are labeled in this section just caudal to the inferior colliculus. A laterally bowed line connecting the trapezoid body (117) and the inferior colliculus would represent in three dimensions the approximate course of the auditory fibers of the lateral lemniscus.

At the caudal pole of the red nucleus (214) is a group of cerebellothalamic fibers (219). These fibers have cell bodies located in dentate (137, Fig. 48), emboliform (130), and globose (126, Fig. 45) nuclei of the contralateral side; their axons have accumulated in the contralateral superior cerebellar peduncle and crossed in the decussation of the superior cerebellar peduncle (200, Fig. 39) to appear in this section. Some will synapse in the red nucleus (214), while others extend to thalamic nuclei. Ventrally, the medial edge of the crus cerebri (220) is prominent. Note, too, the characteristic position of the oculomotor nerve (217) between the superior cerebellar peduncle (125) and posterior cerebral (407) arteries. An aneurysm of these vessels may, therefore, compress the nerve and affect eye movements. Thrombosis of the posterior medial striate vessels that arise from the posterior cerebral artery can simultaneously affect oculomotor fibers to the ipsilateral muscles and corticospinal fibers in the medial side of the crus cerebri (220) which control contralateral body muscles, and hence produce a crossed paralysis.

Most of the association nuclei of the thalamus are included in this section: the pulvinar (324) overhanging the superior colliculus (210), the large anterior nucleus (326), and

the thin, dorsal lateral nucleus (325), dorsal to the medial nucleus (317) and separated from it by a thin layer of myelinated fibers. Some pale staining intralaminar nuclei are obvious within the internal medullary lamina (339). The mamillothalamic fasciculus (313) is just beginning to turn toward its major termination in the anterior nucleus (326), as will become obvious in the following sections. The column of the fornix (403) is now a massive tract that bisects the hypothalamus sagittally into medial and lateral portions.

10—Medial lemniscus
20—Cuneate fasciculus
21—Cuneate nucleus
23—Vertebral artery
25—Spinal tract of the trigeminal nerve
26—Descending vestibular fibers
103—Pontocerebellar fibers
104—Pontine nuclei
113—Primary fissure
117—Trapezoid body
125—Superior cerebellar artery
127—Inferior vestibular nucleus
128—Medial vestibular nucleus
129—Mesencephalic nucleus and tract of the trigeminal nerve
130—Emboliform nucleus
131—Facial nucleus
132—Superior olivary nucleus
133—Lateral spinothalamic tract
134—Facial fibers
135—Superior vestibular nucleus
136—Lateral lemniscus
143—Lateral vestibular nucleus
209—Inferior colliculus
214—Red nucleus
217—Oculomotor nerve
219—Cerebellothalamic (dentatothalamic) tract
220—Crus cerebri (pes pedunculi)
221—Substantia nigra
302—Optic chiasm
313—Mamillothalamic fasciculus
316—Stria medullaris of the thalamus
317—Medial (dorsal medial) nucleus of the thalamus
318—Fasciculus retroflexus
324—Pulvinar
325—Dorsal lateral nucleus of the thalamus
326—Anterior nucleus of the thalamus
339—Internal medullary lamina of the thalamus
401—Body of the fornix
402—Body of the corpus callosum
403—Column of the fornix
404—Anterior cerebral artery
407—Posterior cerebral artery
410—Crus of the fornix

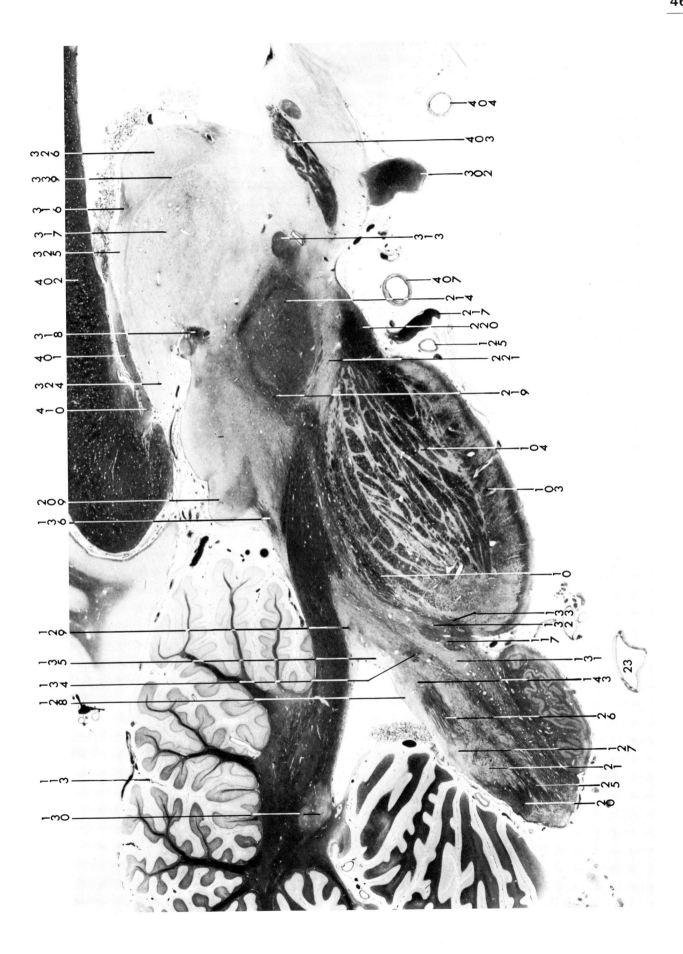

326
339
316
337
325
402

313

407
214
217
220
225
221
29

318
401
324
40

104

103

209
306

10

129

133
123
17

135
131
134
43
128

26

13

27
221
225
20

23

FIGURE 47.

In its course through the spinal cord and brain stem the posterior spinocerebellar tract (24) is visible as an entity that is discrete from adjacent fiber tracts only where it takes an oblique course across the external surface of the spinal trigeminal tract and enters the inferior cerebellar peduncle (28, Fig. 48). Although the posterior spinocerebellar tract is readily distinguished in transverse Figure 9, it also can be appreciated that it would be inconspicuous in sagittal section, such as this figure. Figure 9 also clarifies the dorsal-ventral relationship of the posterior spinocerebellar (24) and spinal trigeminal (25) tracts as seen here in sagittal section. Olivocerebellar fibers (27) interdigitate at nearly right angles with the spinal trigeminal tract and obscure it, just as they do in transverse sections (Fig. 12). These fibers have their origin in the contralateral inferior olive (16), and are here directed dorsally and laterally to become the major constituent of the inferior cerebellar peduncle. Fibers of the facial nerve (134) are sectioned obliquely at the junction of medulla and pons. Since these fibers course ventrally as well as laterally from the internal genu just rostral of the abducens nucleus (121, 122, Figs. 16 and 44), they appear more ventral in this sagittal section than in the previous section.

The superior cerebellar peduncle (211) is massive. Some of the efferent fibers in it have their origin in the emboliform (130) and globose nuclei (126, Fig. 45), but most efferent fibers issue from the dentate nucleus (137, Fig. 50), which lies lateral to the emboliform nucleus. Among the afferent fibers in the superior peduncle, the anterior spinocerebellar tract and those from the mesencephalic trigeminal nucleus are well established. Rostrally, the superior peduncle tapers to a blunt point as the fibers pass medially toward their decussation (200, Fig. 39). Fibers from the contralateral superior cerebellar peduncle help to form the dark mass of cerebellothalamic fibers (219) and cerebellorubral fibers at the caudal end of the red nucleus (214). These cerebellar fibers terminate in the red nucleus or in the thalamus.

Dorsal to the superior cerebellar peduncle, a large segment of the lateral lemniscus (136) is now visible, entering the caudal pole of the inferior colliculus (209). The auditory fibers of the lateral lemniscus are intermixed with spinothalamic (133) and spinotectal fibers here, as indeed they are also in the caudal part of the pontine tegmentum.

Dorsally, in the mesencephalon, the plane of section passes through the lateral slopes of the inferior (209) and superior (210) colliculi. Ventrally there is an appreciable portion of crus cerebri (220) whose fibers can be followed into the pons, where the fibers are labeled jointly corticospinal (118) and corticopontine (124), since they and also corticobulbar fibers cannot be distinguished by the eye.

There is a considerable segment of the fasciculus retroflexus (318) in this section. Immediately ventral to the mamillothalamic tract (313) is a less discrete mass of fibers, the tegmental area H (411), to be discussed later.

10—Medial lemniscus
12—Tela choroidea of the fourth ventricle
16—Inferior olivary nucleus
24—Posterior spinocerebellar tract
25—Spinal tract of the trigeminal nerve
26—Descending vestibular fibers
27—Olivocerebellar tract
33—Anterior spinocerebellar tract
105—Fourth ventricle
118—Corticospinal fibers
124—Corticopontine fibers
125—Superior cerebellar artery
127—Inferior vestibular nucleus
129—Mesencephalic nucleus and tract of the trigeminal nerve
130—Emboliform nucleus
133—Lateral spinothalamic tract
134—Facial fibers
135—Superior vestibular nucleus
136—Lateral lemniscus
210—Superior colliculus
211—Superior cerebellar peduncle
217—Oculomotor nerve
219—Cerebellothalamic (dentato-thalamic) tract
220—Crus cerebri (pes pedunculi)
305—Anterior commissure
313—Mamillothalamic fasciculus
317—Medial (dorsal medial) nucleus of the thalamus
318—Fasciculus retroflexus
324—Pulvinar
325—Dorsal lateral nucleus of the thalamus
327—Lateral hypothalamus
400—Splenium of the corpus callosum
403—Column of the fornix
404—Anterior cerebral artery
406—Body of the lateral ventricle
407—Posterior cerebral artery
408—Tela choroidea of the lateral ventricle
410—Crus of the fornix
411—Tegmental area H

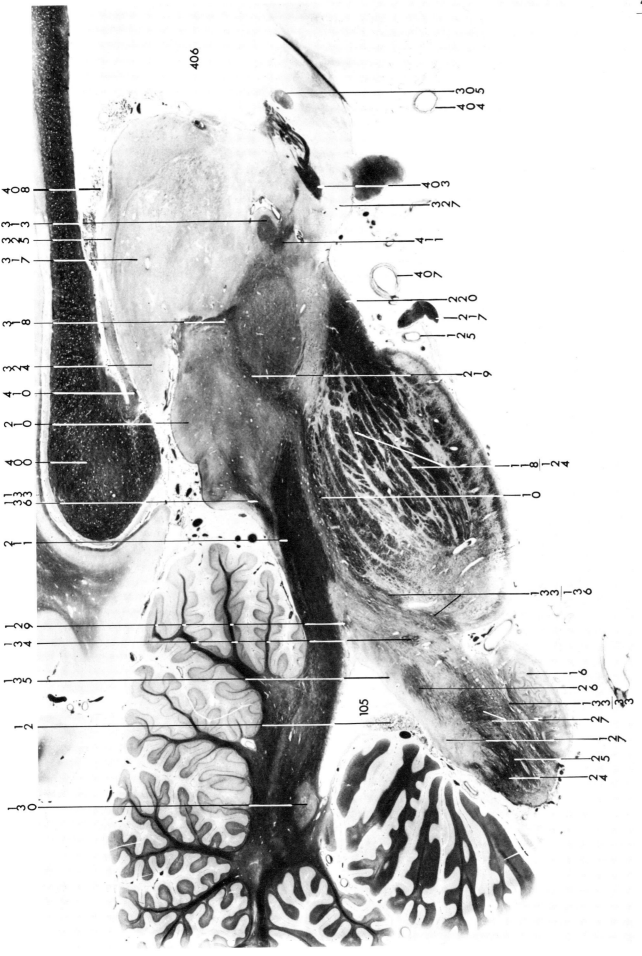

406

105

FIGURE 48.

Only a small segment of the lateral edge of the column of the fornix (403) remains in the section. The area ventral to it is therefore the lateral hypothalamic area. Optic fibers in this section, which have now traversed the optic chiasm, are properly designated the optic tract (328).

Major ascending fiber tracts constitute that portion of the medulla still present in Figure 48. Most dorsal is a segment of the inferior cerebellar peduncle (28). Ventral to it is a longer segment of the spinal trigeminal tract (25), partly obscured by intersecting olivocerebellar fibers (27) which pass through it to enter the peduncle. The lighter and most ventral fibers are ascending anterior spinocerebellar (33) and lateral spinothalamic (133) fibers.

The spinal trigeminal tract (25) can be followed rostrally to its origin from the entering root fibers of the trigeminal nerve (138). In addition to these root fibers, which descend as the spinal trigeminal tract to terminate in the spinal trigeminal nucleus, others ascend and synapse in the superior sensory trigeminal nucleus (141). Still other root fibers (and these are peripheral processes of primary neurons) ascend as the mesencephalic tract (129), along which are scattered the perikarya which form the mesencephalic nucleus of the trigeminal nerve. Finally, in the trigeminal root (138) there are axons of motor neurons whose cell bodies constitute the motor nucleus of the trigeminal nerve (140).

The juxtarestiform body (139) appears as if it were a rostral continuation of the inferior cerebellar peduncle, although at the transverse level of the juxtarestiform body (Fig. 15) it is actually medial to the peduncle; the juxtarestiform body (139) is sometimes considered a medial component of the inferior cerebellar peduncle or restiform body. Juxtarestiform fibers convey impulses to and from the cerebellum. Among afferent fibers are the central processes of primary vestibular neurons and the secondary vestibulocerebellar or nucleocerebellar fibers which arise in the inferior and medial vestibular nuclei (127 and 128, Fig. 45). Efferent fibers that arise in both fastigial nuclei (120, Fig. 44) synapse in vestibular and reticular nuclei in the tegmentum

of the pons and in the medulla. Some of these fibers, called the uncinate fasciculus, arch dorsally and laterally over the superior cerebellar peduncle (211) while still within the cerebellum to gain access to the juxtarestiform body; others enter the juxtarestiform body directly on the medial side of the inferior peduncle. *Leader 138* passes through the fibers of the facial nerve just before they leave the brain stem at the caudal border of the pons.

In the lateral edge of the inferior colliculus is a group of myelinated fibers which form the brachium of the inferior colliculus (222). Most of the fibers of this brachium have cell bodies in the inferior colliculus, but a few proceed directly from perikarya in the trapezoid body, lateral lemniscus, and superior olive into the brachium. The auditory fibers in the brachium of the inferior colliculus can be followed in subsequent sections to their synapse in the medial geniculate nucleus of the thalamus (333, Fig. 53).

The mamillothalamic fasciculus (313) is beginning to curve rostrally in this section. Its caudal edge is not distinct from quite different fibers which belong to the tegmental fields. Tegmental area H_2 (412) contains fibers which originate chiefly in the globus pallidus (421, Fig. 57). The fibers achieve their position in field H_2 either by passing through the internal capsule or by going around its rostral edge, as can be seen in the following sections and in Figures 31 to 35 of the transverse series. These fibers of tegmental area H_2 course caudally and medially into tegmental area H (411). Within area H most of the fibers become recurrent and pass rostrally into H_1, while others continue caudally. Although the course of these fibers in the three planes of space is difficult to follow in two dimensional sections, a concept of their course will be developed in the following legends.

10—Medial lemniscus
23—Vertebral artery
25—Spinal tract of the trigeminal nerve
27—Olivocerebellar tract
28—Inferior cerebellar peduncle
33—Anterior spinocerebellar tract
103—Pontocerebellar fibers
104—Pontine nuclei
113—Primary fissure
125—Superior cerebellar artery
127—Inferior vestibular nucleus
129—Mesencephalic nucleus and tract of the trigeminal nerve
133—Lateral spinothalamic tract
136—Lateral lemniscus
137—Dentate nucleus
138—Trigeminal fibers
139—Juxtarestiform body
140—Motor trigeminal nucleus
141—Superior sensory trigeminal nucleus
211—Superior cerebellar peduncle
219—Cerebellothalamic (dentatothalamic) tract
220—Crus cerebri (pes pedunculi)
221—Substantia nigra
222—Brachium of the inferior colliculus
313—Mamillothalamic fasciculus
317—Medial (dorsal medial) nucleus of the thalamus
318—Fasciculus retroflexus
324—Pulvinar
325—Dorsal lateral nucleus of the thalamus
326—Anterior nucleus of the thalamus
328—Optic tract
402—Body of the corpus callosum
403—Column of the fornix
404—Anterior cerebral artery
407—Posterior cerebral artery
411—Tegmental area H
412—Tegmental area H_2

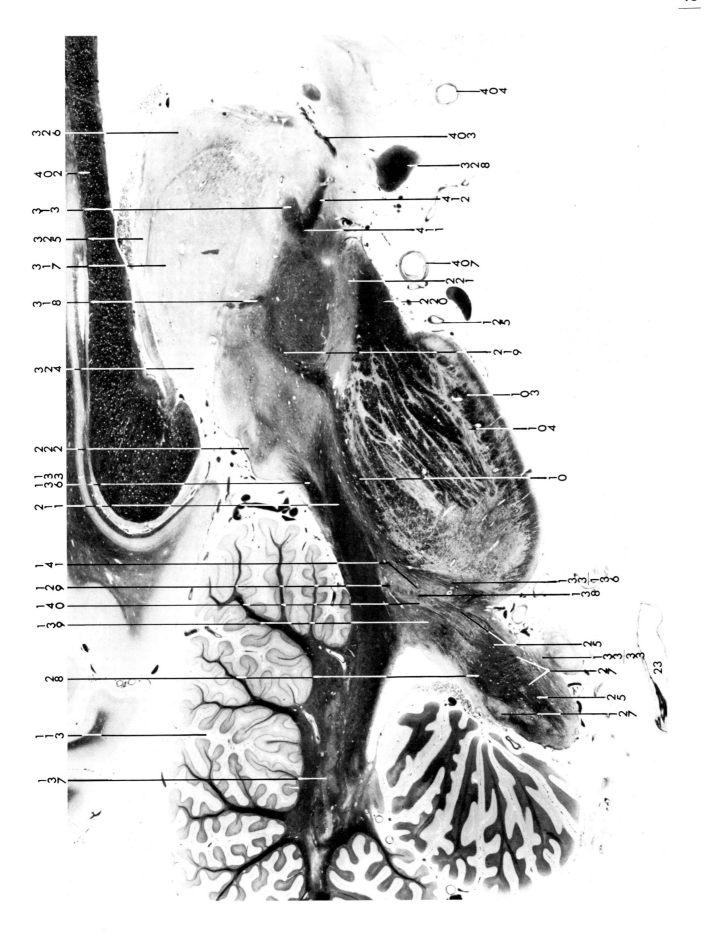

FIGURE 49.

The inferior cerebellar peduncle (28) and the spinal trigeminal (25) and olivocerebellar (27) tracts are more distinct from each other here than in Figure 48. In addition, oblique segments of the afferent and efferent fibers which constitute the juxtarestiform body (139) can now be traced in a recurrent course into the cerebellum. Although not visible in these figures, some fibers arch across the superior cerebellar peduncle (211, Fig. 48) as the uncinate fasciculus, while others take a more direct and ventral course into the cerebellum.

The major source of the superior cerebellar peduncle—the dentate nucleus (137)—now bulks larger in the cerebellar white matter, but only a short segment of peduncle itself (211) is included in the plane of the section. Rostral to it are the intermingled fibers of the lateral spinothalamic tract (133) and the lateral lemniscus (136). Figures 46 to 48 showed oblique segments of the two ends of the tracts caudally and rostrally in the pons; here the two ends appear as one as they curve around the lateral side of the superior cerebellar peduncle. Figure 19 clarifies the anatomical relations of the peduncle and lateral lemniscus. Notice also the relations of the medial lemniscus (10) and lateral lemniscus (136) to each other, both here and in Figure 19.

In the mesencephalon, the plane of section is lateral to the inferior colliculus and so slices the brachium of the inferior colliculus (222) close to its major origin in the inferior colliculus. These auditory fibers can be traced laterally in the following figures to their synapse in the medial geniculate nucleus (333, Fig. 54). The lateral spinothalamic tract (133), ventral to the brachium, can be followed toward its termination in the posterolateral ventral thalamic nucleus (336, Fig. 55).

A section of the anterior ventral nucleus (329) appears at the rostral end of the thalamus. While not sharply delimited in Weigert

sections, the nucleus is characterized by the large number of myelinated fibers, which give it a mottled aspect; these fibers enter or leave the internal capsule as the anterior thalamic peduncle.

The mamillothalamic tract (313) is now an entity distinct from tegmental area H (411) and tegmental area H$_2$ (412). Some fibers of tegmental area H are just beginning to curve rostrally immediately behind the mamillothalamic tract; this will become obvious in the next section.

What is labeled here is actually the posterior forceps of the anterior commissure (305). Since it extends posteriorly as well as laterally, the commissure is relatively much further caudal in this section than it is in the midsagittal Figure 39.

The fornix is also diverging rather more sharply from the midline and from its opposite member in the left hemisphere; this portion of the tract, as it curves down into the temporal lobe, is called the crus of the fornix (410). The body of the fornix is the more rostral part, where it courses close to its contralateral partner and where it is suspended from the corpus callosum by the septum pellucidum.

The optic tract (328) is sectioned obliquely, since the fibers extend laterally and caudally so as to come into ventral relation with the crus cerebri (220, Fig. 52). Compare this relation here in Figure 49 with that in Figures 50 to 54.

10—Medial lemniscus
12—Tela choroidea of the fourth ventricle
25—Spinal tract of the trigeminal nerve
27—Olivocerebellar tract
28—Inferior cerebellar peduncle
105—Fourth ventricle
118—Corticospinal fibers
124—Corticopontine fibers
133—Lateral spinothalamic tract
136—Lateral lemniscus
139—Juxtarestiform body
211—Superior cerebellar peduncle
214—Red nucleus
219—Cerebellothalamic (dentatothalamic) tract
220—Crus cerebri (pes pedunculi)
222—Brachium of the inferior colliculus
305—Anterior commissure
313—Mamillothalamic fasciculus
317—Medial (dorsal medial) nucleus of the thalamus
324—Pulvinar
325—Dorsal lateral nucleus of the thalamus
328—Optic tract
329—Anterior ventral nucleus of the thalamus
400—Splenium of the corpus callosum
404—Anterior cerebral artery
406—Body of the lateral ventricle
407—Posterior cerebral artery
408—Tela choroidea of the lateral ventricle
410—Crus of the fornix
411—Tegmental area H
412—Tegmental area H$_2$

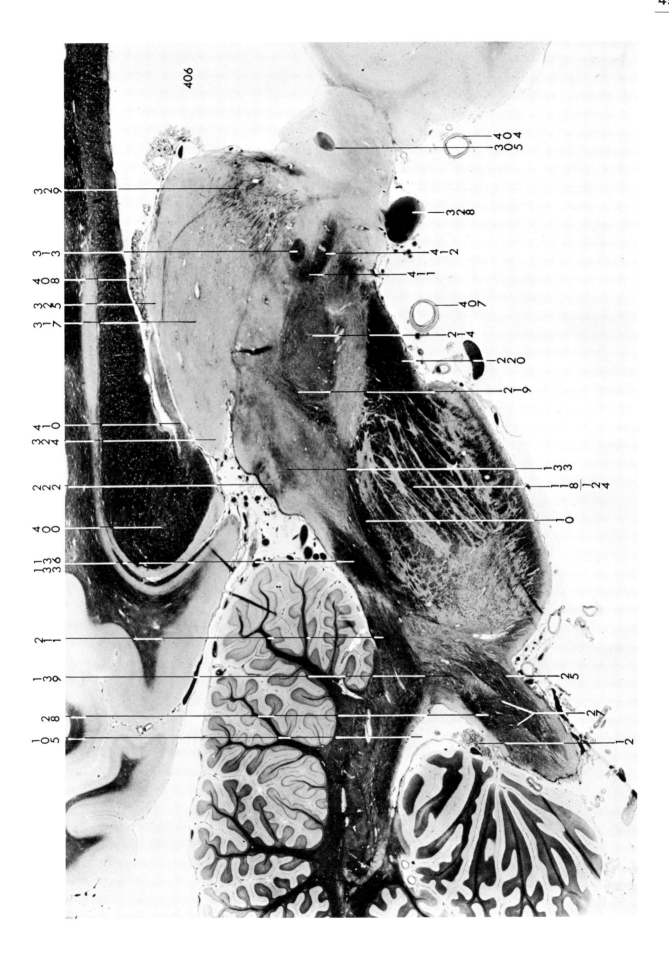

FIGURE 50.

The outstanding feature in the caudal end of the section is the great sweep of the inferior cerebellar peduncle (28) into the cerebellum, where it arches dorsally over the dentate nucleus (137) and the emergent superior cerebellar peduncle (211, Fig. 48). Figure 14 shows the course and relations of the inferior peduncle to the dentate nucleus and the superior peduncle in transverse section at this level.

In the caudal area of the pons, pontine nuclei are greatly reduced and the pontocerebellar fibers are converging into a compact mass, the middle cerebellar peduncle (142). The two trigeminal nerves are the landmarks which separate the middle cerebellar peduncle from the basilar pons. Pontocerebellar fibers between the two trigeminal nerves are in the basilar pons; when the same axons extend dorsally and laterally beyond either nerve they constitute the middle cerebellar peduncle.

Rostrally, the large mass of fibers that extend into the pons from the crus cerebri (220) is made up of corticospinal, corticobulbar, and corticopontine fibers. Impulses propagated in the corticopontine fibers reach the cerebellum via the middle cerebellar peduncle, after traversing a synapse in the pontine nuclei. In turn, impulses modified somehow by the cerebellum are projected back to the cerebrum via the superior cerebellar peduncle, thalamus, and internal capsule.

Fibers of the medial lemniscus (10) and the lateral spinothalamic tract (133) are labeled in the tegmentum of the mesencephalon. It is well to locate the plane of this section in Figures 20 and 21 and review the position and relations of these tracts. Both tracts follow an oblique semicircular course around the lateral side of the superior cerebellar peduncle. The spinothalamic tract (and auditory fibers) swing around first, and the medial lemniscus follows the course of the pain and temperature fibers.

The brachium of the superior colliculus (223) is prominent ventral to the overhanging pulvinar (324). Axons in this brachium have perikarya in the ganglion layer of the retina and mediate reflexes initiated by light. In Figures 49 and 48, fibers of the brachium are not labeled, since they have begun to diverge toward their terminations in the pretectal area and the superior colliculus. In Figures 51 to 57, the brachium can be followed antidromically toward its divergence from the optic tract.

Only the lateral edge of the anterior thalamic nucleus (326) is included in the section, but the dorsal course of the mamillothalamic tract (313) toward the nucleus through the caudal edge of the anterior ventral nucleus (329) is evident. Figure 36 shows that the tract spreads out as it approaches the lateral and ventral aspect of the anterior nucleus.

The recurrent course of some of the fibers in tegmental areas is now apparent. Many axons in this myelinated area have their origin in the lentiform nucleus and either pass through the internal capsule or pass around its medial edge as a tract called the ansa lenticularis (413). Since these fibers pass around and accumulate on the medial side of the internal capsule, the ansa appears in serial sagittal sections before the internal capsule. Using the optic tract (328) as a landmark, note that the ansa (here) occupies the same relative position the internal capsule (418) does in Figure 53. Once they have either coursed through or around the internal capsule, the fibers extend caudally and medially in tegmental area H_2 (412) to enter tegmental area H (411). From area H some fibers continue caudally, to synapse in the prerubral nucleus and the pontopeduncular nucleus. The pontopeduncular nucleus is situated in the light triangular area of reticular formation between the inferior colliculus and the superior cerebellar peduncle in Figures 46 and 47. The legend to Figure 21 locates the nucleus in transverse sections.

However, most fibers leave area H in a recurrent course and run rostrally to synapse in the intermediate ventral (337, Fig. 55), anterior ventral (329), and central (330) nuclei in the thalamus. These recurrent fibers form tegmental area H_1 (414), sometimes called the thalamic fasciculus. The nucleus between tegmental areas H_1 and H_2 is the zona incerta (415).

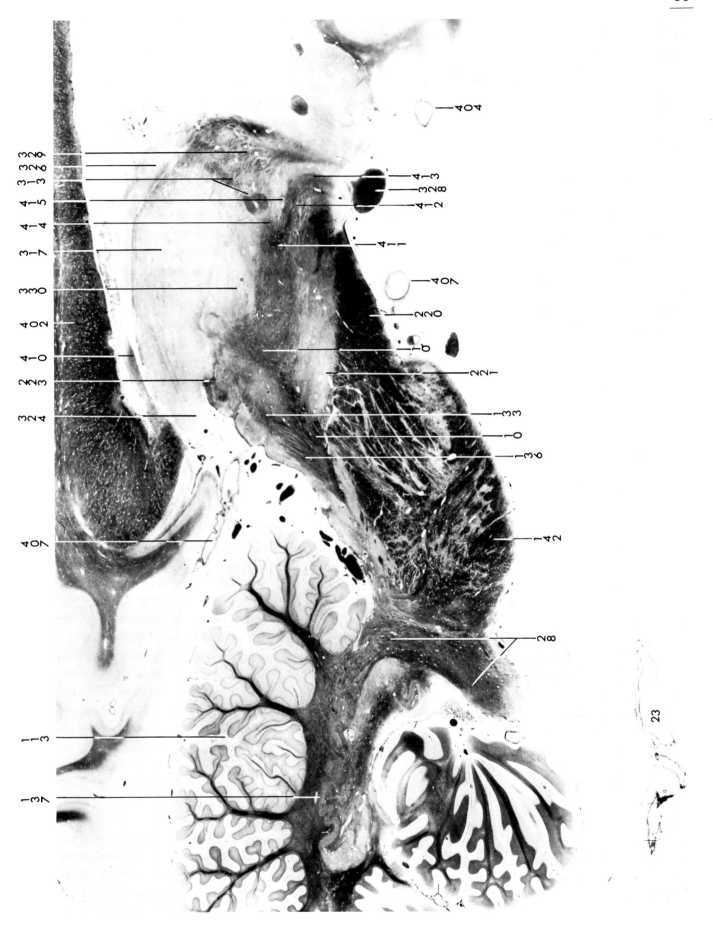

404

339
332

313

438
428

412

415

414

411

317

330

407

402

220

410

223

8

221

324

313

10

316

407

142

13

28

23

17

137

FIGURE 51.

Figure 51 includes the central segment of the inferior cerebellar peduncle (28) as it swings out of the medulla and arches dorsally over the dentate nucleus (137). This peduncle is not visible in the undissected brain, since the pontocerebellar fibers which constitute the middle cerebellar peduncle (142) cover it as they course upward into the cerebellum; this can be verified in Figure 53 and in Figure 14 of the transverse series.

Dorsal to the optic tract, many more of the fibers in the ansa lenticularis (413) can now be followed into tegmental area H₂ (412) and beyond, into tegmental areas H (411) and H₁ (414), all four forming a nearly horizontal S. Many fibers of tegmental area H₁ (414) terminate in the anterior ventral nucleus of the thalamus (329) and the intermediate ventral, from which tracts extend to the frontal cerebral cortex. This establishes the possibility for a modulating feedback upon the cortex from the corpus striatum. Other fibers of area H (411) course caudalward. Pallidosubthalamic and strionigral fibers traverse the internal capsule and synapse without entering the tegmental fields. The *white* segment of leader 331 ends on the strionigral fibers which are also visible in Figure 29 between the subthalamus and the substantia nigra.

The largest nucleus of the intralaminar group of thalamic nuclei, aptly named the central nucleus (330), is delimited by fibers of the internal medullary lamina of the thalamus. Ventral to this nucleus are cerebellothalamic fibers (219), whose course as the superior cerebellar peduncle has been identified in more medial sections. It terminates by dividing into anterior (404) and middle cerebral arteries. The medially directed anterior cerebral was already present in Figure 39. Mingled with the cerebellothalamic fibers are fibers which have emerged from tegmental area H and are directed to the prerubral area and pedunculopontine nucleus.

Caudal to the central nucleus is the medial lemniscus, which is labeled at three places (10). In the midbrain the lateral spinothalamic tract (133) is dorsal to the medial lemniscus, but this is more readily appreciated in Figure 22. It has been the experience of surgeons who have cut the lateral spinothalamic tract at the level of the mesencephalon (mesencephalic tractotomy) that there is a loss of pain and temperature sensibility in the contralateral side of the face as well as of the body. These observations suggest that the ventral central trigeminal tract is associated with the lateral spinothalamic tract in the rostral mesencephalon (Fig. 22). In the myelinated area caudal to the central nucleus, however, all three groups of fibers are intermingled—trigeminothalamic (31) and lateral spinothalamic (133) tracts and the medial lemniscus (10).

The mamillothalamic tract (313) is now a large tract which spreads out near its termination. Because it enters the anterior nucleus of the thalamus from its lateral side, the nucleus is not visible in this figure.

The posterior cerebral artery (407), which takes a semicircular course around the mesencephalon, is sectioned both dorsal and ventral to it. Dorsally, branches are extending caudalward toward their distribution in the medial side of the occipital lobe of the cerebrum. The internal carotid artery (416) is now included in the figure.

10—Medial lemniscus
12—Tela choroidea of the fourth ventricle
28—Inferior cerebellar peduncle
31—Ventral central trigeminal tract
104—Pontine nuclei
133—Lateral spinothalamic tract
136—Lateral lemniscus
144—Dorsal cochlear nucleus
219—Cerebellothalamic (dentatothalamic) tract
220—Crus cerebri (pes pedunculi)
222—Brachium of the inferior colliculus
223—Brachium of the superior colliculus
305—Anterior commissure
313—Mamillothalamic fasciculus
324—Pulvinar
328—Optic tract
329—Anterior ventral nucleus of the thalamus
330—Central (centromedian) nucleus
331—Subthalamic nucleus
400—Splenium of the corpus callosum
404—Anterior cerebral artery
406—Body of the lateral ventricle
407—Posterior cerebral artery
408—Tela choroidea of the lateral ventricle
410—Crus of the fornix
411—Tegmental area H
412—Tegmental area H₂
413—Ansa lenticularis
414—Tegmental area H₁
415—Zona incerta
416—Internal carotid artery

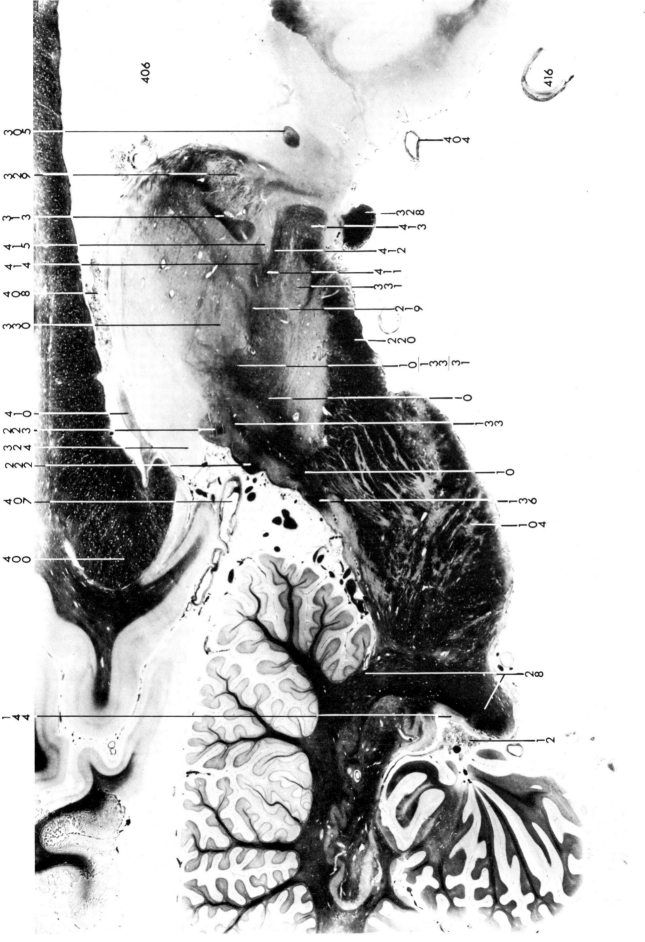

FIGURE 52.

The major constituent of the pons in this section is the middle cerebellar peduncle (142), although a little of the basilar pons, with its nuclei and tracts, is included rostrally.

The entire rostrocaudal extent of the crus cerebri (220) is sectioned, so that these fibers can be followed antidromically from the pons through the crus cerebri into the internal capsule. They appear to be concealed temporarily by the ansa lenticularis (413). Rostral to the ansa, however, these dark fibers again are sectioned and labeled the posterior limb of the internal capsule (418). The corticospinal, corticobulbar, and corticopontine fibers, which constitute the crus cerebri, are also major constituents of the internal capsule. Other important components of the internal capsule, not present in the crus, are the reciprocal connections of thalamus and cerebral cortex. The optic tract (328) is the superficial landmark which delimits the crus cerebri caudally from the internal capsule rostrally.

Ventral to the central nucleus (330) is the slightly darker posteromedial ventral nucleus (332), in which terminate most of the trigeminothalamic fibers mediating pain, temperature, and touch.

Ventral to these two nuclei is a large area of myelinated fibers labeled the cerebellothalamic tract (219) (although the area has the other constituents discussed earlier), which is continuous with tegmental area H₁ (414). Area H₂ (412) appears to end somewhat abruptly caudally because the fibers course medially into area H in Figure 51. In area H, some of the fibers become recurrent and reappear in Figure 52 as components of tegmental area H₁.

At the rostral end of the figure the plane of section begins to include the medial edge of the head of the caudate nucleus (417), which projects into the lateral ventricle (406).

The superior cerebellar artery (125) is sectioned both dorsal and ventral to the mesencephalon. It follows a semicircular path parallel to the posterior cerebral artery (407) around the mesencephalon to reach the upper surface of the cerebellum and parts of the superior and middle cerebellar peduncles.

10—Medial lemniscus
28—Inferior cerebellar peduncle
31—Ventral central trigeminal tract
125—Superior cerebellar artery
133—Lateral spinothalamic tract
137—Dentate nucleus
142—Middle cerebellar peduncle
219—Cerebellothalamic (dentatothalamic) tract
220—Crus cerebri (pes pedunculi)
221—Substantia nigra
222—Brachium of the inferior colliculus
223—Brachium of the superior colliculus
313—Mamillothalamic fasciculus
324—Pulvinar
328—Optic tract
329—Anterior ventral nucleus of the thalamus
330—Central (centromedian) nucleus
331—Subthalamic nucleus
332—Posteromedial ventral nucleus of the thalamus
404—Anterior cerebral artery
407—Posterior cerebral artery
412—Tegmental area H₂
413—Ansa lenticularis
414—Tegmental area H₁
415—Zona incerta
416—Internal carotid artery
417—Head of the caudate nucleus
418—Posterior limb of the internal capsule

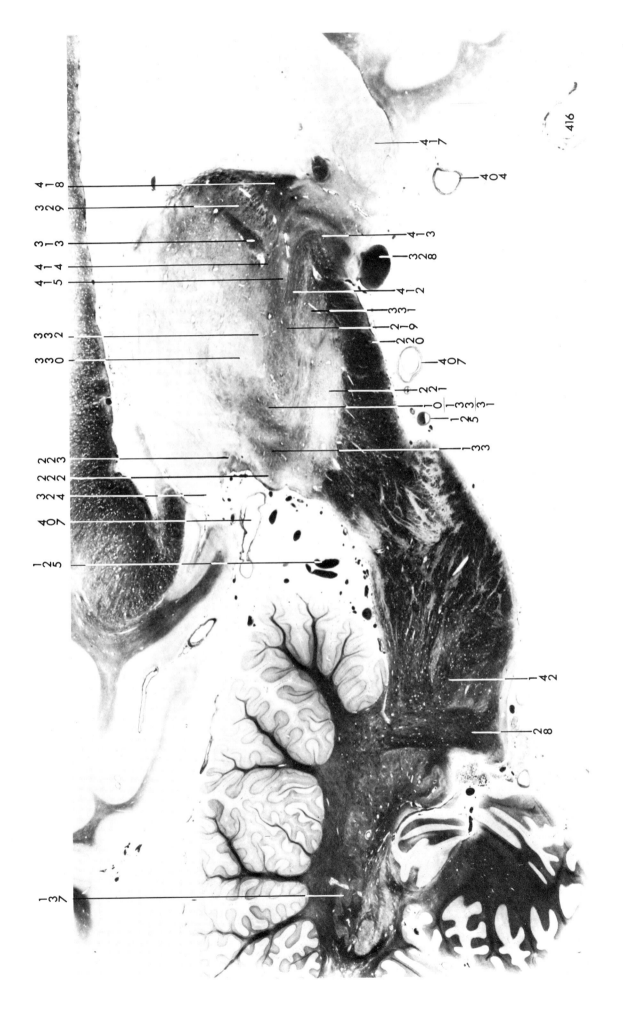

416

FIGURE 53.

A large segment of the dentate nucleus (137) occupies the cerebellar white matter. The inferior cerebellar peduncle (28) arches over it dorsally, and this peduncle is, in turn, covered by the middle cerebellar peduncle (142), which extends caudally and dorsally from the pons into the cerebellum. The segment of the dorsal cochlear nucleus (144) is larger than that included in Figures 51 and 52, but it is never as obvious as it is in transverse section (Fig. 13). Immediately adjacent, the tela choroidea (12) fills the lateral recess of the fourth ventricle. The lateral recess tapers into the lateral foramen just beyond the plane of this section. This foramen is bounded both rostrally and ventrally by the inferior cerebellar peduncle, although the immediate ventral boundary is, of course, the dorsal cochlear nucleus. The tela choroidea ordinarily extends through this foramen, so that some cerebrospinal fluid is secreted directly into the subarachnoid space as well as into the fourth ventricle.

The medial edge of the medial geniculate nucleus (333) is now included in the figure, ventral to the overhanging pulvinar. Most of the fibers ventral to it are auditory fibers of the brachium of the inferior colliculus which synapse in the medial geniculate nucleus; rostral to it are intermingled fibers of general somatic sensibility—medial lemniscus (10), lateral spinothalamic tract (133), and ventral central trigeminal tract (31). Presumably, the more rostral of the fibers in this myelinated mass are trigeminothalamic fibers ending, or about to end, in the posteromedial ventral nucleus (332). Dorsal to the medial geniculate nucleus is the brachium of the superior colliculus, extending medially to synapse in the superior colliculus and in the pretectal area (210 and 218, Fig. 45).

The continuity of the internal capsule (418) and the crus cerebri (220) is established. The ansa lenticularis (413) is cut in cross section be-

cause its fibers are extending medially around the internal capsule; dorsal to the internal capsule, the tegmental area H₂ (412) is prominent, but the continuity between the ansa and tegmental field H₂ is no longer visible. Strionigral fibers are a compact bundle between the subthalamus (331) and substantia nigra (221).

Along the rostral and ventral curvature of the dorsal thalamus the external medullary lamina (334) separates the reticular nuclei (340) from the rest of the thalamus. Caudally these reticular nuclei are continuous with the zona incerta (415).

The uncus (420) appears as an isolated island of gray matter ventral to the optic tract (328) and crus cerebri.

Small segments of anteromedial striate vessels (unlabeled) can be followed dorsal to the anterior cerebral artery (404), from which they arise, into the ventral part of the head of the caudate nucleus (417). Anteromedial striate vessels also supply the anterior limb of the internal capsule, but this not visible in this material. However, in Figure 38 the proximity of the anterior limb of the internal capsule (423), head of the caudate nucleus (417), and nearby anterior cerebral artery (404) suggests this actuality.

10—Medial lemniscus
12—Tela choroidea of the fourth ventricle
28—Inferior cerebellar peduncle
31—Ventral central trigeminal tract
113—Primary fissure
125—Superior cerebellar artery
133—Lateral spinothalamic tract
144—Dorsal cochlear nucleus
219—Cerebellothalamic (dentatothalamic) tract
223—Brachium of the superior colliculus
305—Anterior commissure
324—Pulvinar
328—Optic tract
330—Central (centromedian) nucleus
331—Subthalamic nucleus
332—Posteromedial ventral nucleus of the thalamus
333—Medial geniculate nucleus
334—External medullary lamina of the thalamus
339—Internal medullary lamina of the thalamus
340—Reticular nuclei of the thalamus
400—Splenium of the corpus callosum
404—Anterior cerebral artery
406—Body of the lateral ventricle
407—Posterior cerebral artery
408—Tela choroidea of the lateral ventricle
410—Crus of the fornix
412—Tegmental area H₂
413—Ansa lenticularis
414—Tegmental area H₁
415—Zona incerta
416—Internal carotid artery
417—Head of the caudate nucleus
418—Posterior limb of the internal capsule
420—Uncus

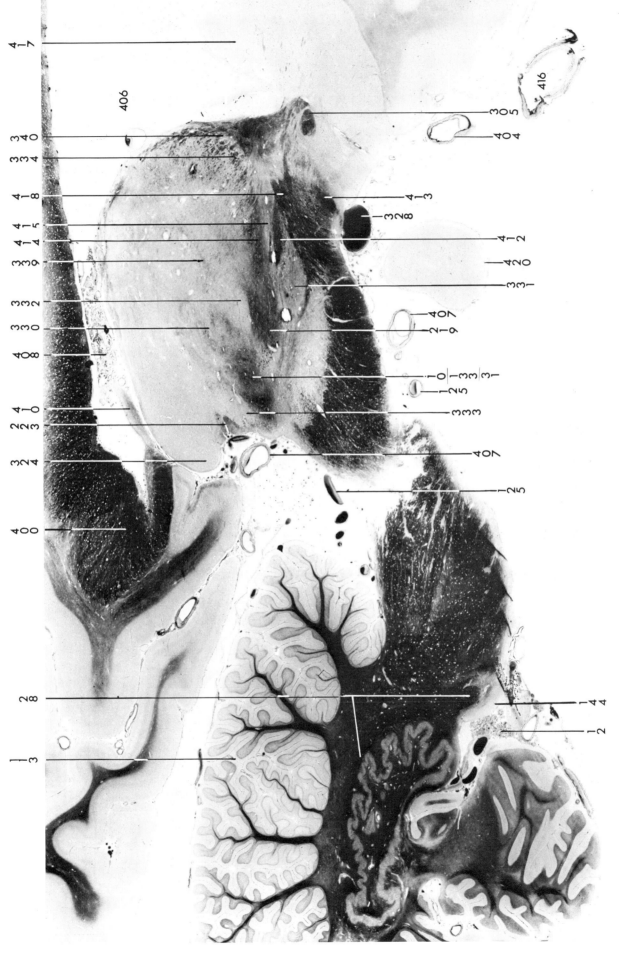

47

406

340

334

4—8

44—5

34—4

339

332

330

48

24—0

223

324

40

28

1—3

305

404

4—3

328

4—2

420

331

407

2—9

1—0 | 331

1—25

333

407

25

1—4

1—2

416

FIGURE 54.

In Figure 54, the cerebellum and pons appear detached from the rest of the brain. Two labeled sections of the superior cerebellar artery (125) dorsal and ventral to the brain stem can now be imaginatively connected into a vessel encircling the mesencephalon to reach the distribution its name indicates. The posterior lateral nucleus (335) makes its first appearance dorsally in the thalamus. It contains few myelinated fibers, and therefore appears paler than the surrounding thalamic nuclei. It is an associational nucleus, with cortical connections in the superior parietal lobule.

Major changes involve the corpus striatum and the internal capsule. The head of the caudate nucleus (417) has been present in previous sections, but the lentiform nucleus is making an initial appearance. This two part nucleus is irregularly conical, with its base lateral and its apex medial. The putamen is the basal portion of the conical lentiform nucleus, while the globus pallidus forms the medial apex. It is the globus pallidus (421) which, therefore, is included first in serial sagittal sections in proceeding from medial to lateral.

The two major portions of the internal capsule, the anterior (423) and posterior (418) limbs, are both present. The internal capsule actually is a large fan-shaped mass of fibers tilted dorsolaterally from the sagittal plane. Medially and ventrally, the fibers of the capsule converge to form the crus cerebri (220). This fan of fibers is also curved, with the concavity directed laterally. The lentiform nucleus occupies this concavity. The posterior limb of the internal capsule (418) is that part which appears in this section between the globus pallidus (421) of the lentiform nucleus and the thalamus. The anterior limb (423) lies between the globus pallidus and the caudate nucleus (417). The genu (422) of the internal capsule is the somewhat poorly delimited

portion of the internal capsule between the anterior and posterior limbs. However, in horizontal section the genu is quite distinct. The posterior forceps of the anterior commissure (305) is ventral to the globus pallidus, and it maintains this position almost to its termination in the temporal lobe. The ansa lenticularis (413), which takes origin from the globus pallidus, is also ventral to it. Note the close relation of the ansa lenticularis to the optic tract (328) and to the anterior commissure (305).

The section includes the origin of the middle cerebral artery (428), one of the two terminal branches of the internal carotid artery (416). The other terminal branch, the anterior cerebral artery, has been present in previous figures. One may visualize the three vessels as a T-shaped arrangement, with the internal carotid artery being the upright of the T; the anterior cerebral artery is the medial half of the cross bar of the T, while the middle cerebral artery is the lateral half. Thus, in following figures the middle cerebral will be present.

The anterior choroidal artery (425) is the slender vessel which can be followed almost to its origin from the middle cerebral artery. In the other direction, it is pointed toward the optic tract (328) which it pierces; additional, unlabeled segments of the anterior choroidal artery occur immediately dorsal to the optic tract in the posterior limb of the internal capsule (418). It is here easy to visualize that the anterior choroidal artery supplies the ventral part of the posterior limb of the internal capsule, the globus pallidus and optic tract. Its close relation to the uncus of the temporal lobe makes it also a "logical" source of blood to the hippocampus and amygdaloid nucleus. Its length, slenderness, and superficial position make it vulnerable to vascular accidents, which result in hemiplegia, hemianesthesia, and hemianopia.

Among the small vessels parallel and dorsal

to the anterior choroidal artery may be one of the direct branches of the internal carotid which supply blood to the genu of the internal capsule.

10—Medial lemniscus
28—Inferior cerebellar peduncle
31—Ventral central trigeminal tract
125—Superior cerebellar artery
133—Lateral spinothalamic tract
137—Dentate nucleus
142—Middle cerebellar peduncle
219—Cerebellothalamic (dentato-thalamic) tract
220—Crus cerebri (pes pedunculi)
221—Substantia nigra
223—Brachium of the superior colliculus
324—Pulvinar
330—Central (centromedian) nucleus
332—Posteromedial ventral nucleus of the thalamus
333—Medial geniculate nucleus
334—External medullary lamina of the thalamus
335—Posterior lateral nucleus of the thalamus
340—Reticular nuclei of the thalamus
407—Posterior cerebral artery
413—Ansa lenticularis
415—Zona incerta
416—Internal carotid artery
417—Head of the caudate nucleus
418—Posterior limb of the internal capsule
420—Uncus
421—Globus pallidus
422—Genu of the internal capsule
423—Anterior limb of the internal capsule
425—Anterior choroidal artery
428—Middle cerebral artery

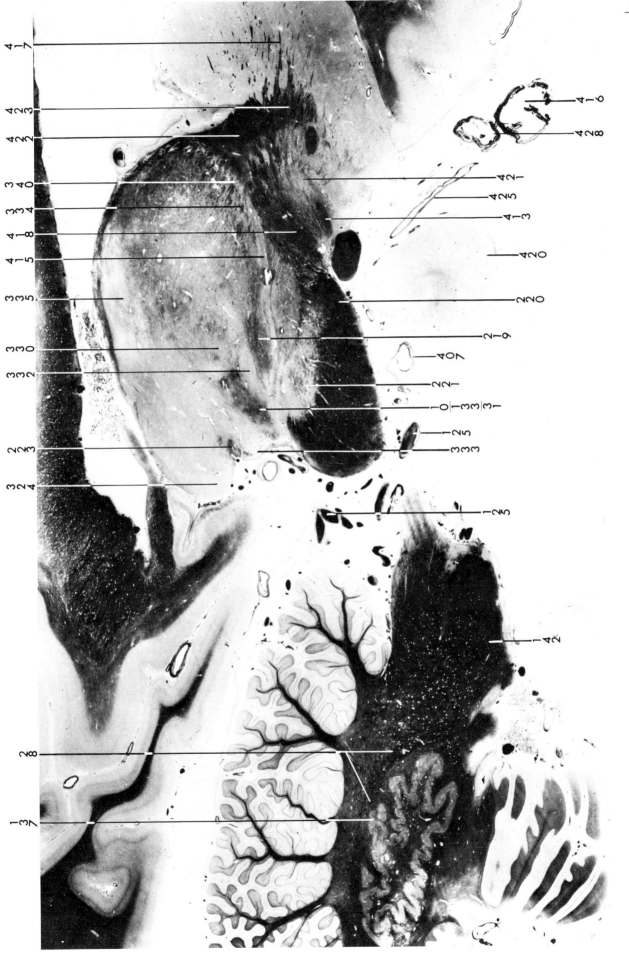

FIGURE 55.

Developments in thalamic structures are of primary interest in this figure. The familiar medial geniculate (333) and posterior lateral (335) nuclei show their greatest areas. The spherical central nucleus, however, is no longer included in the plane of section, and the posterolateral ventral nucleus (336) now occupies a position in this section comparable to that of the posteromedial ventral nucleus (332, Fig. 54). The mass of fibers caudal to the posterolateral ventral nucleus still includes the mingled kinesthetic and tactile fibers of the medial lemniscus (10) and the exteroceptive fibers (pain, temperature, and touch) of the spinothalamic tracts (133). All these terminate chiefly in this posterolateral ventral nucleus. However, this mass of fibers no longer includes the trigeminothalamic fibers, which have by now synapsed in the posteromedial ventral nucleus. The rostral part of the thalamus in this section is largely made up of the anterior ventral (329) and intermediate ventral (337) nuclei. There is no visible boundary between the two.

The mass of fibers ventral to the postero lateral ventral nucleus of the thalamus (336) includes fibers which have been followed rostrally as the superior cerebellar peduncle but which are here more properly labeled the cerebellothalamic tract (219). This tract terminates in the intermediate ventral (337), anterior ventral (329), and small intralaminar nuclei. Also extending rostrally in this myelinated area are pallidothalamic fibers which occupied tegmental fields H and H_1 in more medial sections. Pallidothalamic fibers synapse largely in the anterior ventral, the intermediate ventral, and central (330, Fig. 54) nuclei.

The posterior horn (424) is the subdivision of the lateral ventricle which extends into the occipital lobe of the cerebrum.

10—Medial lemniscus
12—Tela choroidea of the fourth ventricle
113—Primary fissure
133—Lateral spinothalamic tract
219—Cerebellothalamic (dentato-thalamic) tract
220—Crus cerebri (pes pedunculi)
223—Brachium of the superior colliculus
305—Anterior commissure
328—Optic tract
329—Anterior ventral nucleus of the thalamus
331—Subthalamic nucleus
333—Medial geniculate nucleus
334—External medullary lamina of the thalamus
335—Posterior lateral nucleus of the thalamus
336—Posterolateral ventral nucleus of the thalamus
337—Intermediate ventral nucleus of the thalamus
340—Reticular nuclei of the thalamus
400—Splenium of the corpus callosum
406—Body of the lateral ventricle
407—Posterior cerebral artery
408—Tela choroidea of the lateral ventricle
410—Crus of the fornix
413—Ansa lenticularis
420—Uncus
421—Globus pallidus
422—Genu of the internal capsule
423—Anterior limb of the internal capsule
424—Posterior horn of the lateral ventricle
428—Middle cerebral artery

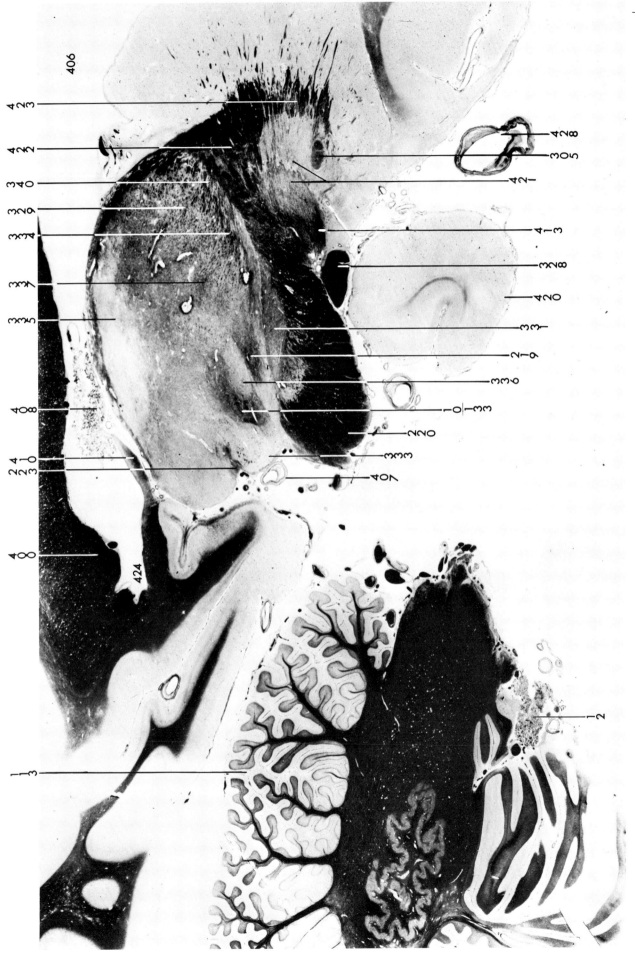

FIGURE 56.

There is little in Figure 56 which is not visible in either the preceding or following sections, but its omission would make the changes between the two unduly abrupt.

The posterolateral fissure (100) is once again quite distinct, as it was in Figure 39 and many following figures; it separates the flocculus (145) and the nodulus (106, Fig. 39), collectively the floccular-nodular lobe, from the corpus cerebelli, which constitutes the rest of the cerebellum. The other major fissure of the cerebellum, the primary fissure (113), divides the corpus cerebelli into anterior and posterior lobes, whose anatomic relations to the primary fissure are indicated by their names. Ventral to the flocculus there is a tuft of the tela choroidea of the fourth ventricle (12) which has protruded through the lateral foramen into the subarachnoid space.

Changes in the diencephalon and what little remains of the rostral mesencephalon are too slight to warrant comment. The optic tract (328) is now closely applied to the crus cerebri (220) which it encircles to terminate, in great part, in the lateral geniculate nucleus (338, Fig. 58). This nucleus occupies a position in more lateral sections comparable to the position of the medial geniculate (333) in this section. Because the semicircular course of the optic tract between the optic chiasm and the lateral geniculate body is roughly in the horizontal plane, each section of the tract starting with Figure 48 is progressively further caudal. Sections of the anterior choroidal artery (425) occur in the optic tract and within the medial segment of the globus pallidus (421) just dorsal to it. It is easy to visualize the distribution of such vessels into the ventral part of the posterior limb of the internal capsule (418) and globus pallidus (421).

The posterior limb of the internal capsule (418) is sectioned not only dorsal to the globus pallidus but also along the dorsal perimeter of the thalamus. Locating the plane of this section in Figure 34 clarifies the inclusion of these fibers dorsal to the thalamus here.

A quick review of the preceding and following figures will show that sections of the caudate nucleus begin with the head (417, Fig. 52) as a small ventral mass in the floor of the lateral ventricle (406) and that it thereafter progressively expands over the internal capsule (423). Initially, in embryologic development, the putamen and caudate are one nuclear mass. However, as axons of neurons located in the cerebral cortex grow into and through this mass (to form the anterior limb of the internal capsule) they partially subdivide the single mass into the head of the caudate nucleus and the putamen. Because the ventral part of this nuclear mass is not invaded by fibers of the internal capsule, there is nothing to mark the transition from medial, caudate nucleus to the lateral, putamen. Thus, on an embryologic basis, it is illogical to group the putamen and globus pallidus together as the lentiform nucleus. Furthermore, "lentiform" does not seem to suggest its true shape.

10—Medial lemniscus
12—Tela choroidea of the fourth ventricle
100—Posterolateral fissure
133—Lateral spinothalamic tract
137—Dentate nucleus
142—Middle cerebellar peduncle
145—Flocculus
219—Cerebellothalamic (dentatothalamic) tract
223—Brachium of the superior colliculus
324—Pulvinar
329—Anterior ventral nucleus of the thalamus
331—Subthalamic nucleus
333—Medial geniculate nucleus
334—External medullary lamina of the thalamus
336—Posterolateral ventral nucleus of the thalamus
337—Intermediate ventral nucleus of the thalamus
340—Reticular nuclei of the thalamus
407—Posterior cerebral artery
413—Ansa lenticularis
415—Zona incerta
417—Head of the caudate nucleus
418—Posterior limb of the internal capsule
419—Putamen
420—Uncus
425—Anterior choroidal artery
429—Internal medullary lamina of the globus pallidus

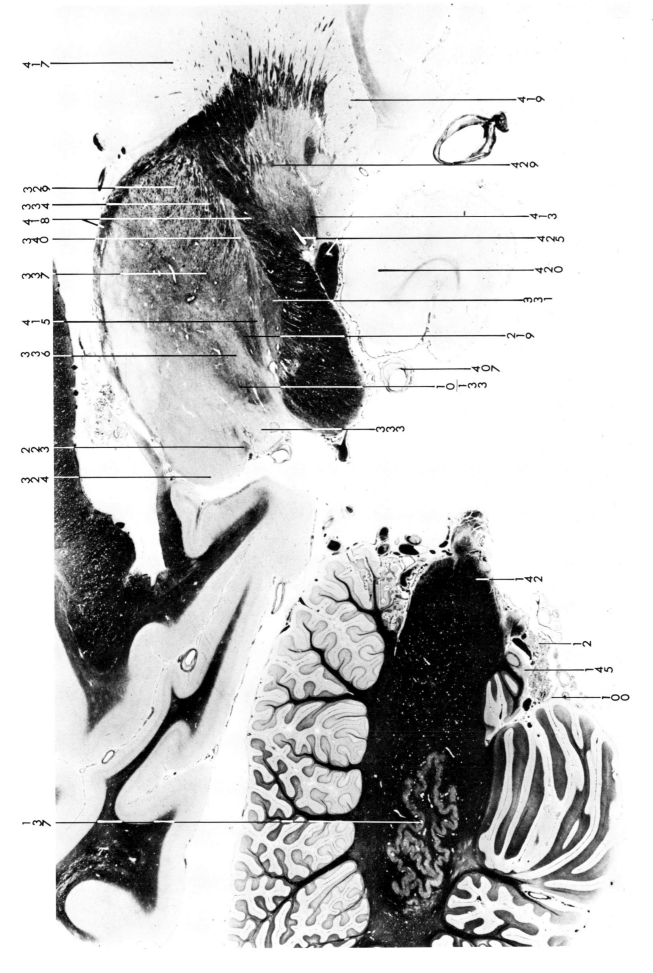

FIGURE 57.

The plane of figure 57 is sufficiently lateral that the uncus (420) and the amygdaloid nucleus (427) appear continuous with the rest of the temporal lobe. The close proximity of the amygdaloid nucleus to the putamen (419), the globus pallidus (421), and the claustrum (457, Fig. 36) accounts for their having been grouped together as basal ganglia. On a functional basis, the association of the amygdaloid nucleus with the corpus striatum is inappropriate. The two sections of the posterior cerebral artery (407) seen in preceding figures (Figs. 50 to 56) dorsal and ventral to the crus cerebri (220) are now joined in this section at the apex of the vessel's semicircular path around the mesencephalon.

The area of the thalamus as a whole is appreciably smaller, as are the medial geniculate nucleus (333) and the pulvinar (324) which are parts of the thalamus. Probably little, if any, of the anterior ventral nucleus remains, the heavily myelinated portion of the thalamus being the intermediate ventral nucleus (337). Considerably larger segments of the posterior limb (418), anterior limb (423), and genu (422) of the internal capsule are now included. The area of the head of the caudate nucleus (417) is notably increased, and the body of the caudate nucleus (435) is present dorsal to the thalamus, as it curves along its lateral aspect toward the temporal lobe. Both the medial and lateral portions of the globus pallidus (421), separated by the internal medullary lamina (429), are included. Reference to sagittal plane 57 in Figure 36 shows that this is possible. The continuity of the ansa lenticularis (413) and this internal medullary lamina is apparent.

In the fissure between the temporal and frontal lobes dorsal to the middle cerebral artery (428) there are two sections of the several anterolateral striate arteries (434) which take origin from the middle cerebral artery. These are major sources of blood to the dorsal part of the posterior limb of the internal capsule, lateral side of the globus pallidus (421), and putamen (419). Transverse sections, such as Figure 34, show that the internal capsule slants dorsolaterally from the sagittal plane, while anterolateral striate vessels (434) have a nearly vertical course through the globus pallidus, so that they necessarily enter the dorsal reaches of the internal capsule. Unlabeled sections of the anterior choroidal artery can be seen here (Fig. 57) in the medial part of the globus pallidus and the ventral part of the internal capsule; a large branch is labeled (425) in the optic tract (328).

The rostral tip of the inferior horn (426) of the lateral ventricle now appears in the temporal lobe immediately caudal to the amygdaloid nucleus (427). Ventral to the inferior horn is the hippocampus (432). On the ventricular surface of the hippocampus is a thin layer of myelinated fibers which is called the alveus (433) of the hippocampus, since these fibers take origin from neurons in the hippocampus. In succeeding sections (Figs. 58 to 62) is is possible to trace the physical continuity of the alveus, via the fimbria of the hippocampus (440, Fig. 62) also known as the fimbria of the fornix, with the crus of the fornix (410), visible here just dorsal to the pulvinar (324) of the thalamus. In preceding sections (Figs. 56 to 45) the crus of the fornix can be traced successively as the body and column of the fornix to the mamillary nucleus. Thus, this fornical system of fibers follows a long circuitous course: it takes origin in and ends on neurons relatively close together. Figure 29 shows this proximity of the hippocampus and the mamillary body. As previously noted, precommissural fibers of the fornix pass rostral of the anterior commissure into the septal area.

The splenium of the corpus callosum (400) no longer has the sharp caudal edge it presented in Figures 39 to 53. After fibers of the corpus callosum cross the midline, the more caudal ones begin to spread out and curve into the occipital lobe of the cerebrum. These caudal fibers in the two hemispheres are collectively called the major forceps (430) of the corpus callosum. The plane of this figure is now sufficiently lateral that one segment of the major forceps is included. Two similar groups of fibers sweep from the rostral end of the corpus callosum into the frontal lobes to form the minor forceps. The corpus callosum is the major physical connection that permits the integration of neural activity of the two cerebral hemispheres.

100—Posterolateral fissure
113—Primary fissure
137—Dentate nucleus
145—Flocculus
220—Crus cerebri (pes pedunculi)
223—Brachium of the superior colliculus
305—Anterior commissure
328—Optic tract
333—Medial geniculate nucleus
335—Posterior lateral nucleus of the thalamus
337—Intermediate ventral nucleus of the thalamus
400—Splenium of the corpus callosum
407—Posterior cerebral artery
408—Tela choroidea of the lateral ventricle
410—Crus of the fornix
413—Ansa lenticularis
418—Posterior limb of the internal capsule
419—Putamen
421—Globus pallidus
422—Genu of the internal capsule
423—Anterior limb of the internal capsule
424—Posterior horn of the lateral ventricle
425—Anterior choroidal artery
426—Inferior horn of the lateral ventricle
427—Amygdaloid nucleus
428—Middle cerebral artery
429—Internal medullary lamina of the globus pallidus
430—Major forceps of the corpus callosum
431—Parahippocampal gyrus (hippocampal gyrus)
432—Hippocampus
433—Alveus
434—Anterolateral striate branches of the middle cerebral artery
435—Body of the caudate nucleus
436—Calcarine fissure

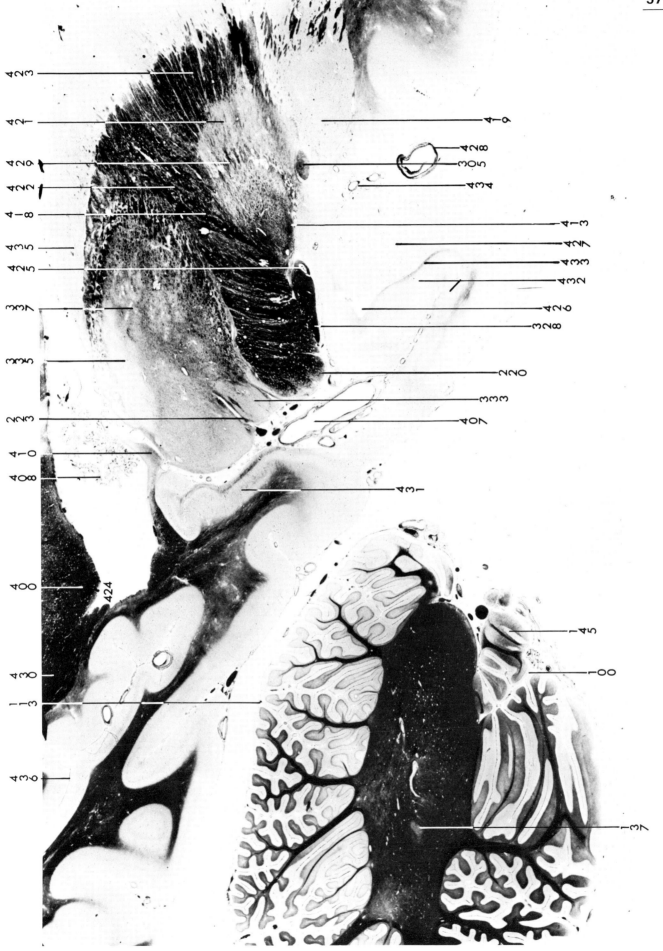

423

421

429

422

418

435

425

337

335

223

410

408

400

424

430

113

436

419

428

305

434

413

427

433

432

426

328

220

333

407

431

145

100

137

FIGURE 58.

There is nothing in the shape and position of the lateral geniculate nucleus (338) to distinguish it from the medial geniculate nucleus in the preceding figures, but it is most indubitably identified by fibers of the optic tract (328) which course around the lateral edge of the crus cerebri and are here seen terminating in the lateral geniculate nucleus. However, fibers originating in the medial geniculate nucleus form the auditory radiations (442) in the triangular area dorsal and rostral of the lateral geniculate nucleus. The auditory radiations then extend rostrally through the retroand sublenticular parts of the internal capsule to terminate in the auditory cortex of the transverse temporal gyri.

Much less of the thalamus is now included in the plane of the section and, correspondingly, more of the internal capsule. Fibers of the posterior limb of the internal capsule (418) slant dorsolaterally and pass to the lateral side of the body of the caudate nucleus (435). Compare with Figure 33.

The tela choroidea (408) largely fills the tip of the inferior horn of the lateral ventricle (426). This portion of the tela choroidea is vascularized chiefly by branches of the anterior choroidal artery (425). Perforating branches of the anterior choroidal artery are prominent in the optic tract and along the internal medullary lamina of the globus pallidus (421). The hippocampal fissure (438), which is formed during embryonic development when the hippocampus rolls inward (laterally), is marked by sections of blood vessels which were originally superficial cortical branches of the anterior choroidal artery in the pia mater. The hippocampus and the tela choroidea receive blood also from a posterior choroidal branch of the posterior cerebral artery (407), but despite this compound supply, the hippocampus is notably susceptible to anoxia.

Several sections of anterolateral striate ves-

sels are present in the lateral fissure (Sylvian fissure) between the middle cerebral artery (428) and the limen of the insula (441) and in the ventral part of the putamen (419). The limen is the ill defined region between the anterior perforated substance rostrally and the ventral part of the insula. If the frontal and temporal lobes of the brain are likened to fingers and thumb, the limen is comparable to the web of the thumb.

100—Posterolateral fissure
145—Flocculus
324—Pulvinar
328—Optic tract
338—Lateral geniculate nucleus
407—Posterior cerebral artery
408—Tela choroidea of the lateral ventricle
417—Head of the caudate nucleus
418—Posterior limb of the internal capsule
425—Anterior choroidal artery
426—Inferior horn of the lateral ventricle
431—Parahippocampal gyrus (hippocampal gyrus)
433—Alveus
435—Body of the caudate nucleus
438—Hippocampal fissure
441—Limen of the insula
442—Auditory radiations

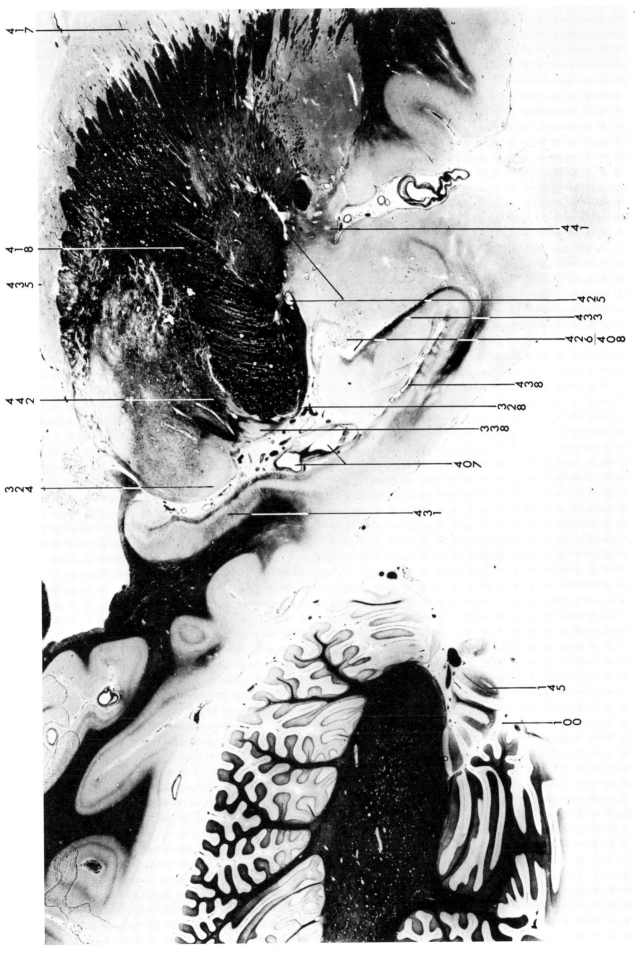

FIGURE 59.

The two thalami, when viewed in three dimensions, are roughly egg-shaped masses arranged at an angle to each other so that they are close together rostrally and diverge caudally. Only the caudal and laterally diverging part of the right thalamus is included in this section. The posterior lateral nucleus (335) and pulvinar (324) appear markedly reduced in size, while the plane of section still transects the medial half of the lateral geniculate nucleus (338). Many fibers of the optic tract are terminating in this nucleus. It will be recalled that other fibers of the tract, which mediate light reflexes, bypass the lateral geniculate nucleus at about this plane to form the brachium of the superior colliculus, which terminates in the pretectal area (218, Fig. 45) and superior colliculus (210, Fig. 47). The course of this brachium (223) can be seen distinctly in Figures 57 to 50. Medial to this, fibers of the brachium begin to diverge and become indistinct, although visible.

The segment of the internal capsule included in the figure is now quite large. The anterior limb of the internal capsule (423) is identified by the strands of gray matter extending through it and making the putamen (419) and head of the caudate nucleus (417) parts of one nuclear mass, the neostriatum. The posterior limb of the capsule (418) and the genu, which lack gray matter, are uniformly dark and compact. All these fibers extend beyond the confines of the corpus striatum and thalamus into cerebral white matter as the corona radiata. Part of the corona radiata (446, Fig. 60) is seen dorsal to the globus pallidus (421) at the very edge of this figure. Here the fibers are cut close to where they interdigitate with transversely oriented fibers of the corpus callosum. The interdigitation is dorsal and lateral to the body of the lateral ventricle (Fig. 37).

The segment of the putamen (419) included in the section is now increased, but not yet to its greatest size. Since the putamen is the base of a roughly conical lentiform nucleus whose apex is the globus pallidus (421), most of the putamen lies lateral to the greater part of the posterior limb of the internal capsule which is visible in this figure. If one imaginatively superimposed the putamen of Figure 62 upon this figure, the parts of the posterior limb not concealed by the lentiform nucleus would be sublenticular or retrolenticular, depending upon their spatial relation to the lentiform nucleus.

Actually, only the retrolenticular part is present in Figure 59; it contains the geniculotemporal or auditory radiations (442) and reciprocal fibers to the medial geniculate nucleus. There may be a few fibers of the optic radiations in the retrolenticular internal capsule, but most of them issue from the lateral geniculate nucleus (338) lateral to this figure. The optic radiations extend caudally along the lateral side of the posterior horn of the lateral ventricle, and terminate in occipital cortex, which forms the banks of the calcarine fissure (436). The dark stripe of Gennari (unlabeled) in the calcarine cortex adjacent to the fissure is made up of the axonic endings of optic radiations. The sublenticular part of the internal capsule is included later (445, Figs. 61 to 63).

The body and tail of the caudate together is a much elongated, tapering, and recurrent nucleus, shaped roughly like a U lying on its side. One part is in the floor of the body of the lateral ventricle, while the other arm of the U is in the roof of the inferior horn of the lateral ventricle, which is lateral as well as ventral to the first half. The plane of this sagittal section transects the tail of the caudate nucleus (443) where it is becoming recurrent. Note the rapid shift in its position in the following figures.

Immediately ventral to the tela choroidea (408) of the body of the lateral ventricle is the mass of fibers labeled at its dorsal end the crus of the fornix (410), and at its ventral end the fimbria of the hippocampus (440) or fimbria of the fornix. All of these fibers are the same, and the only change is nominal; one name emphasizes the origin of fibers in the hippocampus (432), while the other emphasizes their continuity with the rest of the fornix. The fimbria of the hippocampus is sectioned and labeled (440) at a second place closer to its origin in the rostral end of the hippocampus. These two ends of the fimbria will approach each other (Figs. 60 to 62) and join (Fig. 63). The dentate gyrus is long and slender and extends parallel with, and adjacent to, the fimbria of the hippocampus but only the two ends of this single gyrus are present in this figure.

This figure shows the origin of another of the many anterolateral striate branches (434) from the middle cerebral artery (428). Additional segments of this vessel are shown entering the anterior perforated substance (unlabeled) and in the putamen (419). Anterolateral striate arteries supply blood to the dorsal part of the posterior limb of the internal capsule and to the immediately adjacent portions of the caudate nucleus.

113—Primary fissure
305—Anterior commissure
324—Pulvinar
335—Posterior lateral nucleus of the thalamus
338—Lateral geniculate nucleus
408—Tela choroidea of the lateral ventricle
410—Crus of the fornix
413—Ansa lenticularis
418—Posterior limb of the internal capsule
419—Putamen
421—Globus pallidus
423—Anterior limb of the internal capsule
424—Posterior horn of the lateral ventricle
427—Amygdaloid nucleus
430—Major forceps of the corpus callosum
431—Parahippocampal gyrus (hippocampal gyrus)
432—Hippocampus
433—Alveus
434—Anterolateral striate branches of the middle cerebral artery
436—Calcarine fissure
439—Dentate gyrus
440—Fimbria of the hippocampus
442—Auditory radiations
443—Tail of the caudate nucleus

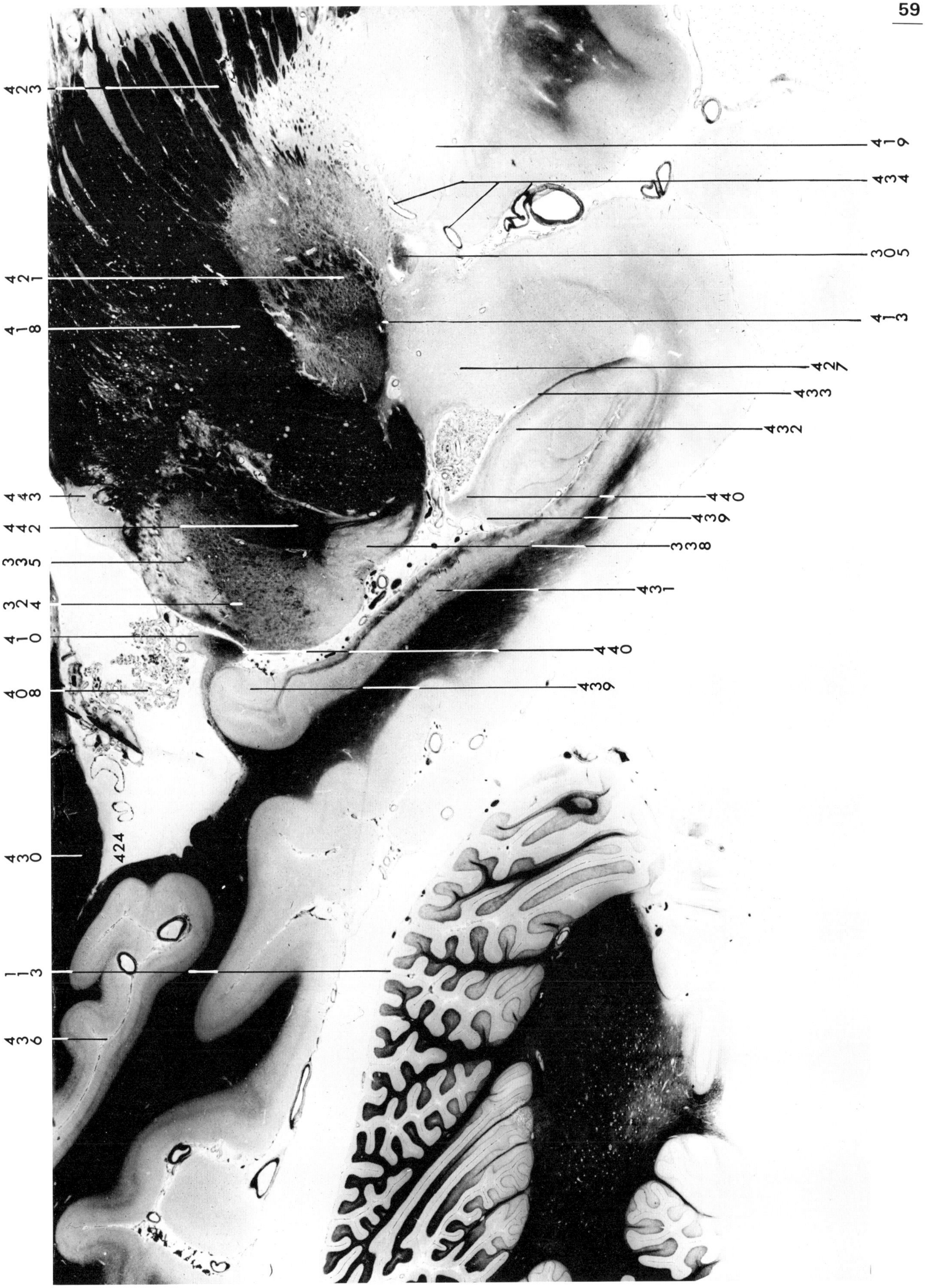
423
421
418
443
442
335
324
410
408
430
424
13
436
419
434
305
413
427
433
432
440
439
338
431
440
439

FIGURE 60.

The lateral geniculate nucleus (338) is here maximal in size, and practically all of its fibers from the optic tract have now entered. The dark halo surrounding the dorsal aspects of the lateral geniculate nucleus contains the geniculocalcarine tract (447) or optic radiations, which is another constituent of the retrolenticular internal capsule (444), along with the auditory radiations. The geniculocalcarine tract is the last link in the pathway conveying impulses initiated by light to the visual area of the cerebrum along the banks of the calcarine fissure (436, Fig. 59). There are also reciprocal fibers in the optic radiations which convey impulses from the occipital cortex to the lateral geniculate nucleus. The calcarine fissure is so deep as to cause a distinct protrusion of the cerebrum into the medial wall of the posterior horn of the lateral ventricle (424). This bulge bears the seemingly irrelevant name of calcar avis (437) or cock's spur.

Ventral to the lateral geniculate nucleus (338), the posterior choroidal branch (449) of the posterior cerebral artery is sectioned. Additional anterolateral striate branches of the middle cerebral artery (428) occupy the fissure between the temporal and frontal lobes. This fissure is now sufficiently deep that it may be designated specifically the lateral fissure of Sylvius.

The globus pallidus (421) is diminished while more of the putamen (419) is included in the plane of section, but the posterior limb of the internal capsule is still widely displayed. Dorsally, the longitudinally sectioned fibers of the corona radiata (446) interdigitate with the transversely oriented and sectioned fibers of the corpus callosum. The tail of the caudate nucleus (443) is diminished in area and has shifted caudally and ventrally, where it is closer to the fimbria of the hippocampus (440) as both fimbria and caudate curve into the temporal lobe.

The anterior commissure (305) (actually the posterior forceps of the anterior commissure) continues to shift caudally as it extends laterally. The extent of this shift is perceived by comparison with the anterior commissure in Figure 39.

338—Lateral geniculate nucleus
418—Posterior limb of the internal capsule
428—Middle cerebral artery
431—Parahippocampal gyrus (hippocampal gyrus)
433—Alveus
437—Calcar avis
438—Hippocampal fissure
439—Dentate gyrus
440—Fimbria of the hippocampus
441—Limen of the insula
443—Tail of the caudate nucleus
444—Retrolenticular part of the internal capsule
446—Corona radiata
449—Posterior choroidal artery

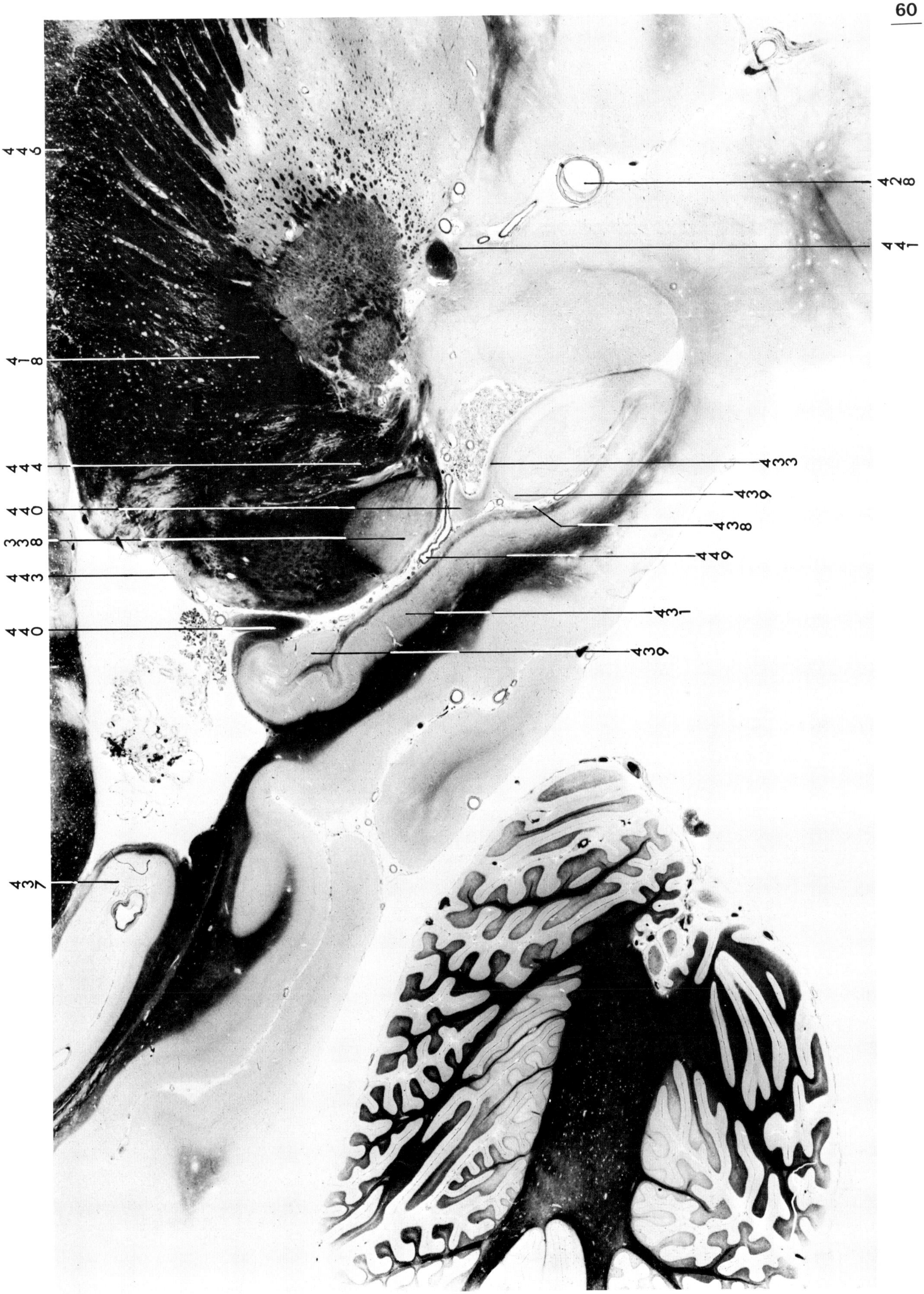
445
418
444
440
338
443
440
437
428
441
433
439
438
449
431
439

FIGURE 61.

Only the most lateral part of the globus pallidus (421) remains, as progressively more of the putamen (419) has been included in the section. The tail of the caudate nucleus (443) is sectioned and labeled twice, once where it has been seen in the previous figure and now, for the first time, through its terminal portion in the roof of the inferior horn of the lateral ventricle (426). This figure shows the proximity of the corpus striatum (419, 421, and 443) and the amygdaloid nucleus (427), which are, with the claustrum, the basal ganglia.

Only a small segment of lateral geniculate nucleus (338) remains, and most of the fibers to and from the nucleus lie in the portions of the posterior limb of the internal capsule called retro- and sublenticular. Those geniculocalcarine fibers (447) which course almost directly caudal to their termination in the calcarine cortex traverse only the retrolenticular portion of the internal capsule (444). Other fibers, which emerge from the rostral aspect of the lateral geniculate body, course rostrolaterally in the roof of the inferior horn of the lateral ventricle for varying distances before they become recurrent, join the direct geniculocalcarine fibers, and extend along the lateral side of the body and posterior horn of the lateral ventricle to the calcarine cortex. These recurrent fibers in the roof of the inferior horn, beneath the lentiform nucleus, are constituents of the sublenticular internal capsule (445). These fibers are called the loop of Archambault and Meyer. This forward extension of the optic radiations is probably associated with the rostral growth of the temporal lobe during development. Whatever the cause, their course accounts for visual deficits associated with lesions in the temporal lobe. The auditory radiations are also important constituents of the retrolenticular internal capsule and, to a slight degree, become sublenticular in their course to the transverse temporal gyri.

The two parts of the fimbria of the hippocampus (440) and the two parts of the dentate gyrus (439) are now appreciably closer to their juncture.

305—Anterior commissure
338—Lateral geniculate nucleus
408—Tela choroidea of the lateral ventricle
418—Posterior limb of the internal capsule
419—Putamen
421—Globus pallidus
426—Inferior horn of the lateral ventricle
427—Amygdaloid nucleus
430—Major forceps of the corpus callosum
432—Hippocampus
433—Alveus
434—Anterolateral striate branches of the middle cerebral artery
437—Calcar avis
438—Hippocampal fissure
439—Dentate gyrus
440—Fimbria of the hippocampus
441—Limen of the insula
443—Tail of the caudate nucleus
444—Retrolenticular part of the internal capsule
445—Sublenticular part of the internal capsule
446—Corona radiata
447—Geniculocalcarine tract
450—Lateral fissure of Sylvius

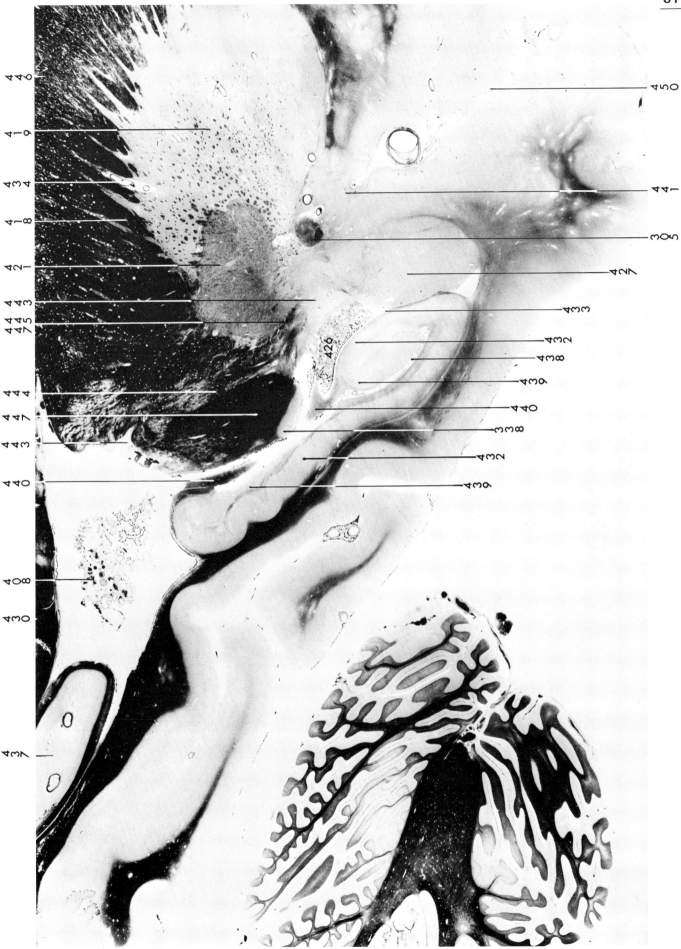

46
49
434
418
421
443
445
447
444
447
443
440
408
430
437

450
441
305
427
433
4332
4338
439
440
3338
4332
439

426

FIGURE 62.

Figure 62 is of interest because the two segments of the fimbria of the hippocampus now are joined, and one can trace the alveus of the hippocampus (433) caudally into it. The dentate gyrus (439) also appears as the long slender gyrus it is. The inferior horn of the lateral ventricle (426) is sectioned twice, once through its rostral portion in the temporal lobe and again at its origin as a ventral extension from the body of the lateral ventricle (406). The hippocampus is a long cylindrical projection into the inferior horn, and one can see the continuity between the two parts of the inferior horn easily only when the plane of section is lateral to the hippocampus. A figurative amputation of the hippocampus would simulate such a lateral section.

The largest possible segment of the putamen is achieved in this section, and the relations of the retro- (444) and sublenticular (445) parts of the internal capsule to the lentiform nucleus are now obvious. The putamen (419) is labeled in its extreme ventral portion to emphasize its continuity with the tail of the caudate nucleus (443).

The posterior part of the anterior commissure (305) is no longer distinctly round in section because the fibers are beginning to diverge toward their destinations. A few of the fibers, which are not continuous in this section with the rest of the commissure, are present dorsal to and within the amygdaloid nucleus (427). They interconnect parts of the limbic system across the midline. Most fibers of the anterior commissure connect neocortical areas of the temporal lobes.

The figure shows both the cortical branches of the middle cerebral artery (428) within the lateral fissure of Sylvius (450) and numerous segments of the anterolateral striate arteries (434) in the rostral part of the putamen.

305—Anterior commissure
406—Body of the lateral ventricle
408—Tela choroidea of the lateral ventricle
418—Posterior limb of the internal capsule
419—Putamen
424—Posterior horn of the lateral ventricle
426—Inferior horn of the lateral ventricle
428—Middle cerebral artery
432—Hippocampus
433—Alveus
434—Anterolateral striate branches of the middle cerebral artery
437—Calcar avis
439—Dentate gyrus
440—Fimbria of the hippocampus
441—Limen of the insula
443—Tail of the caudate nucleus
444—Retrolenticular part of the internal capsule
445—Sublenticular part of the internal capsule
446—Corona radiata
450—Lateral fissure of Sylvius

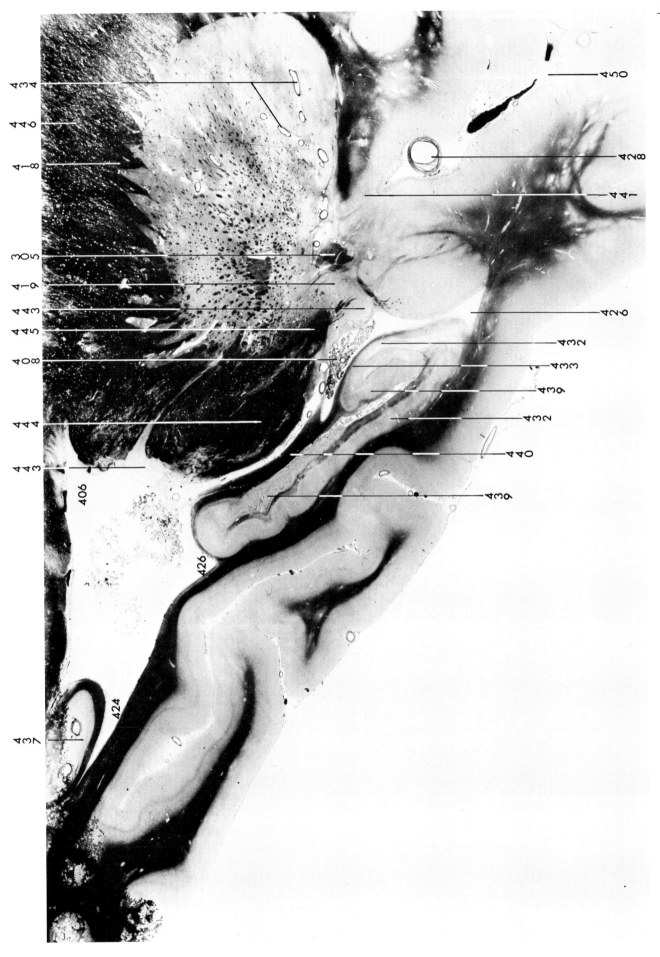

434
446
418

450

428
441

435
419

426

443
445

408

432
433
439
432

444

440

443

439

406

426

437

424

FIGURE 63.

The last section in the atlas is included chiefly because it demonstrates that the tail of the caudate nucleus (443) in the floor of the body of the lateral ventricle does curve ventrally and rostrally to occupy the roof of the inferior horn of the lateral ventricle (426). Since the tail of the caudate does not appear completely continuous in this section, four segments of it are labeled. The tela choroidea of the lateral ventricle (408) is labeled where it occupies the middle portion of the inferior horn of the lateral ventricle, but only the rostral and caudal ends of the inferior horn (426) are labeled.

The vertical course of the anterolateral striate vessels (434) through the putamen (419) toward the dorsal part of the internal capsule is particularly well shown. Ventral to the putamen, from caudal to rostral, are the sublenticular internal capsule (445), the anterior commissure, now much frayed out (305), the external capsule (451), and the uncinate fasciculus (448). As its name suggests, the uncinate fasciculus has a recurrent course from the frontal lobe into the temporal lobe via the limen of the insula (441). Caudally, the small undulations of the fibers in the dentate gyrus (439) just dorsal to the hippocampal fissure (438) mimic the elevations and depressions on the superficial surface that led to its being called the dentate (toothed) gyrus.

305—Anterior commissure
408—Tela choroidea. of the lateral ventricle
419—Putamen
426—Inferior horn of lateral ventricle
427—Amygdaloid nucleus
430—Major forceps of the corpus callosum
432—Hippocampus
433—Alveus
434—Anterolateral striate branches of the middle cerebral artery
437—Calcar avis
438—Hippocampal fissure
439—Dentate gyrus
440—Fimbria of the hippocampus
441—Limen of the insula
443—Tail of the caudate nucleus
444—Retrolenticular part of the internal capsule
445—Sublenticular part of the internal capsule
446—Corona radiata
448—Uncinate fasciculus
450—Lateral fissure of Sylvius
451—External capsule

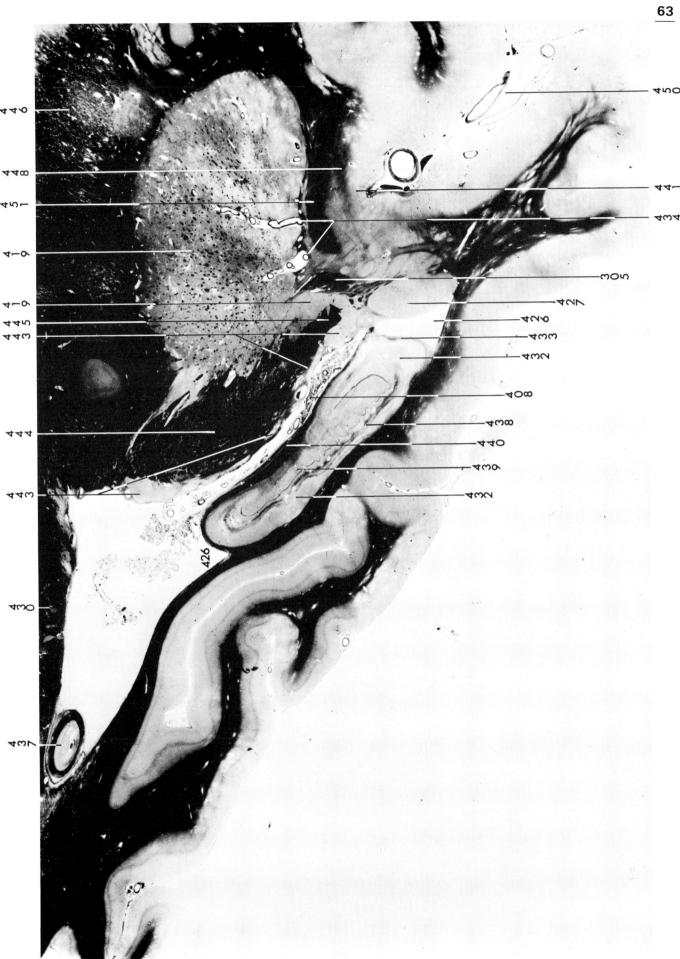

INDEX OF CODE LETTERS AND NUMBERS

CODE LETTERS AND NUMBERS

336—Posterolateral ventral nucleus, thalamus
337—Intermediate ventral nucleus, thalamus
338—Lateral geniculate nucleus
339—Internal medullary lamina, thalamus
340—Reticular nuclei, thalamus
341—Midline nuclei, thalamus
342—Hypothalamic sulcus
343—Hypothalamus
344—Tuber cinereum
345—Interthalamic adhesion (massa intermedia)

Telencephalon

400—Splenium, corpus callosum
401—Body, fornix
402—Body, corpus callosum
403—Column, fornix
404—Anterior cerebral artery
405—Septum pellucidum
406—Body, lateral ventricle
407—Posterior cerebral artery
408—Tela choroidea, lateral ventricle
409—Anteromedial striate artery
410—Crus, fornix
411—Tegmental area H
412—Tegmental area H_2

413—Ansa lenticularis
414—Tegmental area H_1
415—Zona incerta
416—Internal carotid artery
417—Head, caudate nucleus
418—Posterior limb, internal capsule
419—Putamen
420—Uncus
421—Globus pallidus
422—Genu, internal capsule
423—Anterior limb, internal capsule
424—Posterior horn, lateral ventricle
425—Anterior choroidal artery
426—Inferior horn, lateral ventricle
427—Amygdaloid nucleus
428—Middle cerebral artery
429—Internal medullary lamina, globus pallidus
430—Major forceps, corpus callosum
431—Parahippocampal gyrus (hippocampal gyrus)
432—Hippocampus
433—Alveus
434—Anterolateral striate artery
435—Body, caudate nucleus
436—Calcarine fissure

437—Calcar avis
438—Hippocampal fissure
439—Dentate gyrus
440—Fimbria, hippocampus
441—Limen of insula
442—Auditory radiations
443—Tail, caudate nucleus
444—Retrolenticular part, internal capsule
445—Sublenticular part, internal capsule
446—Corona radiata
447—Geniculocalcarine tract
448—Uncinate fasciculus
449—Posterior choroidal artery
450—Lateral fissure, (Sylvius)
451—External capsule
452—Internal cerebral vein
453—Strionigral, pallidotegmental fibers
454—Uncinate gyrus
455—Vena and stria terminalis
456—Extreme capsule
457—Claustrum
458—Insula
459—Fasciculus lenticularis
460—Inferior thalamic peduncle
461—Anterior perforated substance
462—Paraterminal gyrus
463—Subcallosal area

INDEX

Numbers and letters in parentheses denote the structures identified in the plates. The numbers not in parentheses denote the figures, or sequence of figures, in which the structure is visible, even though it may actually be labeled in a preceding or following plate in the sequence.

INDEX

INDEX